ASTHMA ALERT

You have questions:

How can I prevent asthma?
What do the latest studies say?
Do children really outgrow asthma?
What are the special concerns for women who have asthma?
How can I become healthier in an increasingly toxic world?

Dr. Richard Firshein has the answers!

Discover the many factors that can trigger your asthma, and learn how to eliminate or control them to dramatically improve your health. In REVERSING ASTHMA, you'll follow Dr. Firshein through a comprehensive, step-by-step program that uses personalized testing and lifestyle evaluation to target your individual needs. You'll learn how to use diet, environmental adjustments, nutritional supplements, breathing exercises, and mind/body techniques to regain and maintain wellness. This revolutionary program worked for him. It works for nearly all of his patients. Now let it work for you!

PRAISE FROM THE EXPERTS FOR *REVERSING ASTHMA*

"Amazingly informative and filled with vital new knowledge that guides the reader to a healthier, happier life."
— JOSEPH T. MARTORANO, M.D., author of *Beyond Negative Thinking* and founder of Manhattan Biofeedback

"The most comprehensive yet understandable resource I have seen on the natural medicine treatment of asthma. As a physician and lifelong asthma sufferer, Dr. Firshein provides unusually insightful guidance for those wanting to reestablish their health through the artful combination of lifestyle advice, herbs, nutritional supplements, and, when appropriate, drugs."
— JOSEPH E. PIZZORNO, N.D., president of Bastyr University, author of *Total Wellness* and coauthor of *Encyclopedia of Natural Medicine*

"Clear, insightful. It offers new hope and compelling new information for asthma sufferers. A must-read."
— LEWIS KOHL, D.O., chairman of the Emergency Medicine Department, Brookdale University Hospital Medical Center, New York

"Brilliant and innovative! I heartily recommend this book."
— PAUL SORVINO, actor and author of *How to Become a Former Asthmatic*

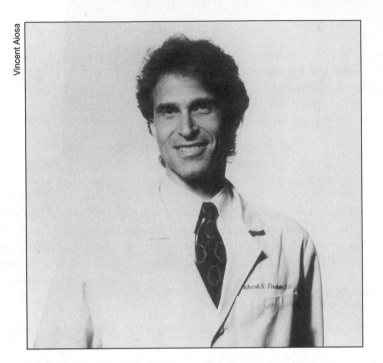

RICHARD N. FIRSHEIN, D.O., is a physician in private practice in New York City. Well known as a lecturer and writer, he is a frequent guest on television and radio, hosts his own weekly call-in radio show, "HouseCalls," and is a contributing editor and columnist for *Psychology Today*. He is an assistant professor of family medicine at the New York College of Osteopathic Medicine, medical director of the Paul Sorvino Asthma Foundation, and recently completed a project evaluating a natural approach to treating cancer through a grant from the Royal Academy of Medicine in Sweden. A leader in the field of alternative medicine, he is the president of Nutraceutical Research, Inc., a corporation dedicated to researching alternative treatments.

REVERSING ASTHMA

BREATHE EASIER WITH
THIS REVOLUTIONARY
NEW ROGRAM

Richard N. Firshein, D.O.

WARNER
WELLNESS

NEW YORK   BOSTON

This book is not intended as a substitute for medical advice of physicians. The reader should regularly consult a physician in all matters relating to his or her health, and particularly in respect of any symptoms that may require diagnosis or medical attention.

Warner Wellness

Warner Books
1271 Avenue of the Americas, New York, NY 10020

Warner Wellness and the Warner Wellness logo are trademarks.

Printed in the United States of America
First Trade Printing: April 1998
10 9 8 7 6

Library of Congress Cataloging-in-Publication Data

Firshein, Richard.
    Reversing asthma : breathe easier with this revolutionary new
    program
        p. cm.
    ISBN 0-446-67363-3
    1. Asthma—Alternative treatment. I. Title.
RC591.F55   1996
616.2'3806—dc20   96-5721
                                                      CIP

Book design and composition by L&G McRee
Illustrations by Robin Lazarus
Cover design by Diane Luger
Cover photo by Craig Aurness/Westlight

*My deepest gratitude
to my parents Sylvia and Michael
for their love, guidance, and wisdom.*

ACKNOWLEDGMENTS

This book could not have been written without the love, support, and commitment of so many people in my life: My deepest appreciation to Randi Arnold, who shares my life and brings special meaning to every day. My good friend Paul Sorvino, whose work with the Paul Sorvino Asthma Foundation has been a constant inspiration. Kris Dahl, my agent, whose enthusiasm and insight have been crucial to the success of this book. Many thanks to my editor, Joann Davis, whose vision recognized the importance of the material and message of this book, and to Colleen Kapklein for her professional guidance and support throughout the second printing. My dedicated staff: Mary Angela Lauricella for her outstanding work, Vadim Kern for his exceptional and wide range of talents, Amy Frankel, who kept my office running smoothly while I was writing this book, and Charlot Rosario. Thanks to Drs. Lewis Kohl, and Jeff Horowitz. Special thanks to Stuart Young, M.D., at Mt. Sinai Hospital for his care and guidance. To Gabe DeSimone of the Good Earth Health Food Stores, Bill Thompson, editor-in-chief of *Natural Health Magazine*, and Owen J. Lipstein, editor-in-chief of *Psychology Today*, for their commitment to Natural

Medicine. Special appreciation to Johan Brohult, M.D., professor of medicine at the Karolinska Institute in Sweden. Together we are researching natural healing substances in the hope that medicine will move increasingly in the direction of nutritional healing. I am particularly grateful to Cathrin Guenther for her extraordinary dedication and commitment, and for teaching me the true meaning of friendship. I want to thank my two brothers, Dan and Steve—both of whom are physicians—along with their wives, Barbara and Joy. A special thanks to Steve and Barbara for giving me a place to rest and recuperate after I was hospitalized at the National Jewish Center in Denver, as well as to the innovative physicians at that clinic. Thanks to the physicians at the New York College of Osteopathic Medicine for all their guidance, in particular the dean, Stanley Schiowitz, D.O., and professors Joe Renders, Gary Ostrow, and Bob Mancini, as well as Abe Jeger, Ph.D., Arnold Nagler, Ph.D., and Bob Cummings, Ph.D. I am grateful to the children, parents, and teachers at P.S. 85 for their participation in research on breathing and asthma, and to Irwin Rappaport, M.D., co-director of the Children's Asthma and Allergy Center at the Cornell Medical Center at New York Hospital. Special thanks to the staff of the Chicago University Library, Fordham University Library, St. John's University Reference Library, Rockefeller University, the New York Public Library, the New York Botanical Garden, the New York Horticultural Society, the American Forestry Association, the Museum of Natural History, Elsevier Science, Pharmacia Diagnostics, and BioReference Laboratories for their assistance in researching material for this book. I want to thank all my patients, whose remarkable healings have inspired me and made our journey together so meaningful. And finally, special thanks to Jill Neimark; without her help each step of the way this book would not exist.

CONTENTS

FOREWORD

by Paul Sorvino

Dr. Richard Firshein is, for me, a twenty-first-century physician with the medical specifications of a Park Avenue primatur and the best abilities and instincts of an ancient healer. Because of his extraordinary treatments and supplements and his wonderful medical care, I am healthier today than I have ever been in my life. That is why I chose him to be medical director of the Paul Sorvino Asthma Foundation. Brilliance aside, he is an extremely caring and wonderful friend, and I believe that empathy and caring are the most important qualities a healer can have.

I first met him through a mutual friend, who told me that Dr. Firshein had suffered from asthma himself and was helped by the breathing exercises I described in my bestselling book *How to Become a Former Asthmatic.* My own suffering with asthma, which began when I was ten years old, ranged from moderate to severe and went on until I was twenty-five. At that age I learned breathing exercises that literally cured me overnight. These exercises, yogic in origin, have worked for many people, including my own son. Dr. Firshein incorporates breathing exercises as part of his Comprehensive Asthma Program.

Together, we have a dream of building children's asthma centers all over the country. We want to spread the word and make it clear that asthma is a defeatable condition. It is a condition, not an actual disease. Over time it can lead to disease, but with the use of breathing exercises and the natural approach outlined in this book, most asthmatics can become asthma-free.

I couldn't have found a greater ally or a better friend than Dr. Richard Firshein in the quest to help asthmatics around the world.

PREFACE

In this groundbreaking book, Dr. Richard Firshein, a leader in the field of alternative medicine, focuses his tremendous energy and commitment on providing you with a new, proven program for the treatment and prevention of a disease which has reached epidemic proportions in our time—Asthma.

Asthma affects fifteen to twenty million people in the United States alone. Worse yet, thousands die unecessarily each year due to this condition. I have worked for the last ten years at Kings County Hospital in New York City, one of the nation's busiest hospitals. There in the emergency department we see about 10,000 patients a year for mild to severe asthma attacks. For people suffering with asthma, the fear of permanent dependence on medications and the ever-possible recurrence of asthmatic attacks significantly diminishes their capacity to enjoy life and to be happy and productive. This has far reaching effects on family and friends as well.

In this book, Dr. Firshein opens for us a new horizon of possibilities, a new future of health, happiness, and productivity. He was inspired by his own horrendous experience with asthma, and the fact that it did not respond to the available medical care. He began with exhaustive research into the disease, examining all possible therapies. This led to his own recovery, repeated successes in his practice, and finally to this book. He has outlined a step-by-step plan for getting asthmatics healthy, without reliance on medications. For some asthmatics, who are probably the minority, medication is an inescapable reality. Yet even for these people, fewer medicines in lower, more tolerable doses may be feasible, placing less stress on their immune systems.

Asthma is not inevitable. Dr. Firshein educates the reader in understanding the many possible triggers that cause the inflammation and congestion in the bronchial passages leading to asthma attacks. He explains how healing and prevention are achieved by his comprehensive approach which includes diet, nutritional supplementation, environmental modification, breathing excercises, and stress reduction. I can tell you that in my own experience, with these clear directions I have turned emergency department regulars into people I see only on the street.

This book is extensively researched, clearly written and filled with helpful information. Dr. Firshein writes with compassion and understanding for those suffering with this condition, and presents you with a new, comprehensive approach that will change your life, while being manageable and easy to implement. It will give you the knowledge and guidance to get started on a path to renewed health and vitality today. Good luck, and enjoy this valuable resource and what it has to offer you.

—LEWIS KOHL, D.O., Chairman of the Emergency
    Medical Department, Brookdale University Hospital
    Medical Center, Brooklyn, New York

CHAPTER ONE

My Story

I remember the shouting of nurses and doctors on that cloudless Tuesday in August 1986. I had been out of the hospital for only a few minutes—standing on the street corner, about to get into my car, profoundly relieved that the previous week's ordeal was over—and now I was being carried back in.

Eight days earlier, I had awakened in the middle of the night struggling to breathe and unable to walk even a few feet. My medicated sprays, which for years had unfailingly given me back my life and magically opened my airways, no longer worked.

So there I was, doing the one thing I had hoped I would never have to do . . . heading straight to the emergency room. For an asthmatic who has been attempting all his life to prove he's a regular guy—that he can play tennis and basketball like the rest of his friends, that he is not somebody standing on the fringes of life unable to visit homes with pets, a smoky restaurant, or the country when flowers and trees are in bloom—a visit to the emergency room is a frightening admission of defeat. For me, it was also the beginning of a merry-go-round of hospitalizations, a life painfully circumscribed by illness.

The moment I was released from the hospital, I stood on the street corner promising myself that I would never get that ill again. I told myself an infection had caused the virtual collapse of my airways.

Like most asthmatics, I was living in a kind of blind alley. So were my nurses and doctors. We had all been laughing and joking when they discharged me. I had no idea how ill I really was. (I later realized that this hospitalization was not an isolated emergency, but the endpoint of a process of deterioration that had taken place over twenty years.) Just then a bus screeched to a stop in front of me and belched out a big exhaust plume. I breathed it in.

Or to be more accurate, I stopped breathing.

Moments later, I was *back* in the emergency room, and the voices of the doctors and nurses had turned to quiet panic. I was instantly hooked to an IV that dripped powerful steroids and drugs into my veins, so potent that I felt I was losing contact with reality. The nurses looked as if they were miles away. I closed my eyes. My breathing had diminished to a truly frightening point: there was no wheeze left. When an asthmatic's breathing is nearly inaudible, it means he has virtually no air in his lungs. At the same time, my heart was thudding and racing, gunned up by the speedlike chemicals infused into my body.

That night I closed my eyes and tried as hard as I could to breathe. I heard the attending physician say, "If his condition continues to deteriorate, we'll have to intubate him." I knew what that meant: intubation is an extremely uncomfortable procedure where a hard, plastic tube is pushed down the trachea, causing one to gag. The tube is hooked up to a machine that forces air into the lungs. I would be, in essence, breathing by machine.

I couldn't stand the thought. I had to keep myself breathing. I took my pulse and, because my heart was racing, forced myself to breathe in for seven beats and out for nine beats. Controlled breathing along with the pulse is a technique I teach my patients today.

I knew a few of the doctors thought I might not make it that night. Now when I look back, I'm astonished at how little any of us understood my illness. I had spent a week in the hospital at a cost of over ten thousand dollars, and they had released me without any sense of how ill I truly was— and without any tools for dealing with my asthma.

The fact was, none of us had an inkling of why I had gotten so sick and what I really needed: a comprehensive program that included purified air, tests for sensitivities to food, a total change of diet, a discharge plan that included breathing exercises and vitamins, a rest from antibiotics and asthma sprays, an exercise program geared to the asthmatic who is short of breath—all the practices and treatments that I use today to reverse the symptoms of asthma and dramatically lessen the need for drugs. In essence, I needed a revolution in lifestyle.

That night I didn't sleep. Hour after hour passed as I sat up in my hospital bed, forcing myself to inhale and exhale, thinking to myself, "This is not how I'm going to die."

Even more important, that was not how I was going to live.

It's incredible. Fifteen million Americans are suffering from asthma, and 4 million of them are under eighteen. The death rate from asthma has more than doubled since 1978. We spend about $6.2 billion on asthma a year. Asthma, along with AIDS, cancer, and tuberculosis, is a chronic disease on the rise the world over. Twenty percent of the American population—fully 40 million people—suffer from some kind of airway disease, whether it's chronic bronchitis, asthma, or emphysema. According to the National Center for Health Statistics, Americans spend $1 billion yearly on asthma medications, and adults with asthma lose about $850 million a year in wages, while parents with asthmatic children lose $1 billion a year by staying home to care for their children.

It's of great concern to me that asthma fatalities, even though they are steadily rising, may be grossly underestimated. A study from the *Journal of the American Medical Association* found that among more than three hundred people who had died of various causes, 6 percent were thought to have died of asthma. The study put the real figure at 16 percent. And nobody talks about deaths that list asthma as a "contributing" factor.

Asthma no longer plays by the rules doctors have used to describe it for the last two thousand years. Doctors always thought that most children outgrow asthma. The truth, at least today, is that the disease steadily worsens or returns in a disturbing majority of cases. A new study conducted by Dutch and American researchers in the Netherlands found that about 75 percent of children with moderate to severe asthma still suffered from the condition by the time they reached their midtwenties. As the author of the study, Dr. Ruurd Van Roorda, stated, "When you have asthma, you always have asthma."

Imagine watching a child suffocate and die in front of you, a boy or girl who has a whole life ahead. This can happen with almost no warning. An asthmatic with a bronchial infection can go from a normal rate of breathing to death in ten minutes, and there have been far too many reported cases of asthmatics found dead with their sprays in their hands. It happens.

How did this illness become so widespread in an era of medical and technological marvels? Why have deaths and suffering steadily increased in spite of major "advances" in treatment of the disease? That's a subject I'll discuss in detail in chapter 3. Suffice it for now to say that our approach to this disease has been woefully inadequate and misguided, our medications have often worsened the condition over the long term, and few of our doctors have developed the kind of comprehensive treatment program that emphasizes *healing* and *prevention.*

Yet this may be the worst *and* the best of times for asthmatics, for change is in the air. In the last year alone, a significant shift in doctors' attitudes has come about. The head of the Allergic Diseases Section of the National Institutes of Health, Dr. Michael A. Kaliner, believes we have entered a whole new era of asthma therapy. The first era, he contends, took place from 1970 to 1990 and focused on control of symptoms. That era relied heavily on drugs that brought symptomatic relief. The mistakes of that approach were so serious that Kaliner publicly blasted doctors for harming patients.

"No asthmatic should die, and if properly treated, very, very few asthmatics would die," he told *The New York Times* in May 1993.

Kaliner called attention to a new era, ushered in only a few years ago, which treats the underlying causes of asthma. Successful treatment focuses on reducing inflammation. Medicine's new fascination with asthma's underlying causes has led to many new avenues of treatment and to new drugs. We are at the dawning of a new era of genetic medicine— an era in which we already have a primitive but fascinating map of all the human genes. We are already beginning to target certain deadly illnesses, such as cystic fibrosis and sickle cell anemia, for genetic therapy. Cystic fibrosis, it turns out, is a complex illness that seems to be regulated by a whole symphony of genes. When it is mild, it can show up as an illness often misdiagnosed as asthma.

Major medical journals, such as *The Lancet,* are now publishing articles investigating the role of antioxidant nutrients like vitamins C and E in easing or perhaps even helping to prevent chronic diseases, from heart problems to cancer. A whole new field of research has opened up in the area of "free-radical" damage and illness, a topic I will explain in this book.

I am pleased to report that new studies in the medical journals *Chest*, *Thorax*, and *Allergy* are now looking at the role of free radicals in asthma.

I approach asthma in a revolutionary fashion, but I can do so only because I have at my fingertips a wide range of sophisticated, high-tech testing procedures that, when combined with innovative alternative treatments, yield effective cures. That's why I'm excited. Our ability to study asthma at the cellular and genetic level is teaching us a great deal about how and why this disease occurs.

As I see it, asthma is actually a result of a disordered metabolism that occurs at the cellular level. Asthma is the disease of a body on red alert, reacting and overreacting to many substances in the environment—and exhausting itself in the process. For instance, as reported in a 1991 study in *Chest*, certain white blood cells are in a permanently activated state in asthmatic patients. Asthma is such a complex disease—the result of an intricate web of inflammatory chemicals in the body—that it takes a fine detective to ferret out each factor and treat it.

After years of working with patients, I've developed a program to diagnose and treat every aspect of the asthmatic's life—not just his or her lungs. I make sure to clean up the asthmatic's environment—especially the home, which is so often a source of unsuspected allergens. I draw on a vast wealth of nutritional information, the most sophisticated allergy testing, sensitive immunological tests, high doses of vitamins (sometimes intravenously), and alternative methods such as acupuncture, meditation, biofeedback, hypnosis, profound dietary changes, special breathing exercises, and the latest research into new uses of old drugs (such as heparin, which is proving to be a marvelous antiinflammatory substance in small doses). I developed these treatments and techniques through intensive study and self-experimentation, and I have since applied them to my patients with astonishing effectiveness.

My program looks at nutrition, herbs, the environment, and the mind-body connection. I examine the role of yeast, allergies, preservatives, dyes, and toxic chemicals. I also test my patients' homes and offices for molds and toxins and advise them on cleaning up pollutants. I offer innovative treatments—such as intravenous magnesium, which has been documented to work as well as certain drugs in lessening asthma attacks. One study, published in the *Annals of Allergy,* found that intravenous magnesium sulfate given to patients with moderate to severe asthma improved their ability to breathe (as measured by the force and volume of air they were able to exhale). Another study, conducted at the University of Turin, in Italy, found that inhaled magnesium helped reduce the spasms of smooth muscle in the bronchial tubes.

It's truly surprising how profound a difference these gentle but powerful treatments can make. Eighty percent of my asthma patients are now leading active, virtually drug-free lives. If that seems impossible—if you've lived day in, day out wheezing and relying heavily on drugs—listen to the rest of my story. I became very sick before I got well.

My asthma started when I was a little kid. I remember lying alone in my bedroom with my "squeezer," a handheld device that pumped mist and medicine into the lungs. I missed enormous periods of school because of asthma attacks. (What no one knew at the time was that school was probably making me sicker, and it may be harming many asthmatic children today. Consider the impact of inhaling ammonia and chemicals used to clean the floors each day, of tightly shut windows, dust from the chalk, and even the materials used to build the schools. It's only now that, for instance, New York City has recognized that schools may be hazardous to the health. Many schools have been closed down recently because of asbestos problems.)

My problems were not limited to school. At summer

camp, during rainy season, the bunk was moldy, and I'd wake in the middle of the night barely able to breathe. When my parents came up halfway through the summer, I was in such a bad state they took me to an air-conditioned hotel for the afternoon just so I could get some sleep.

In spite of all this suffering, one of the refrains of my childhood was "You don't know how lucky you are." A few decades before, in the "Stone Age" of asthma, children had to submit to thumping devices to force mucus out of the lungs, suction cups placed on the chest, and flannel bindings wrapped tightly around the diaphragm. If these primitive techniques failed to help, the recipe was simple: stay home. Many asthmatic children were forced to be virtual invalids because any foray into the universe outside, particularly school, might trigger an attack.

For me, however, there was a new world of pharmaceutical drugs, drugs that flourished in the 1960s. They're worth taking a close look at, because *none of them are popular today.* They're still listed in the *Physician's Desk Reference,* and you can still get them by prescription, but they've been abandoned by most physicians, in favor of the newest class of drugs, which themselves may eventually be another generation of dinosaurs. Extinct. Some of these new drugs, like the old drugs, often cause uncomfortable side effects and don't do enough to ameliorate the underlying cause of this condition.

Of all the drugs, perhaps the great favorite when I was growing up was a medication called Tedral, which is still available today. It is a blend of two drugs: ephedrine, which opens up constricted bronchial tubes and speeds up the whole nervous system, and phenobarbitol, a strong muscle relaxant and tranquilizer that is intended to counter the side effects of ephedrine. This is ironic at best. Phenobarbitol is known to cause respiratory depression, or a lowering of lung capacity! Besides, consider the paradoxical effect on your nervous system: a drug that speeds you up and slows you down at the same time.

An even more complex chemical cocktail that was popular when I was growing up was known as Marax. This drug contained ephedrine along with theophylline, another bronchial expander and stimulant, and an antihistamine called Atarax, which is known to cause drowsiness. I remember getting up every morning before school and taking liquid Marax. It had a sickeningly sweet taste. Almost immediately, my hands were shaking from the effects of the medication.

Along with drugs, I was fed the conventional wisdom of the day that asthma is largely a psychological illness. If you had trouble breathing, people just thought you were crazy or neurotic. Other chronic diseases, like diabetes or juvenile arthritis, were not labeled psychological.

Yet asthma, like every chronic illness, has a tremendous psychological impact. Imagine somebody putting a pillow over your face and pressing it down so you can't breathe. That's how many of my patients describe an asthma attack, and it engenders intense panic. Panic causes the body to release a flood of fight-or-flight chemicals from the adrenal glands, and that profoundly affects the sufferer's state of well-being.

About the time I got to high school, sprays utilizing a drug called albuterol had become popular—and they still are immensely popular. A single puff and my bronchial tubes seemed to miraculously open and relax. At the time, it seemed the sprays were giving me a new lease on life. My family propelled me into sports, which I loved, but I always had my sprays with me. I remember running around the basketball court during a championship game, shooting a basket, then pulling out my spray and taking a puff—and thinking nothing of it.

Although I began to "feel" well as a teen—as long as I kept my trusty spray in my pocket—I was actually on the road to becoming seriously ill. As I will say time and time again, reliance on drugs alone harms the asthmatic over the long term. I'm not condemning the judicious use of sprays in the proper context, but to rely on drugs as the sole treatment for asthma is a perilous proposition.

Why? Look back with me for a moment. Only a few decades ago, in the 1960s, when our latest brave new arsenal of asthma drugs came to the fore, everybody thought asthma had truly been "banished" forever. These drugs shaped a new generation of asthmatics who relied on their medications freely and easily—and lived "normal" lives. It may have been the worst thing that could have happened to many sufferers. Those drugs allowed smokers to go on smoking, and use their sprays; to go on working in moldy, toxic offices as long as their sprays were in their pockets; to literally bathe themselves in the very toxins that were damaging their lungs, and hardly feel it. In fact, I was one of those asthmatics. I never left home without my spray in my pocket.

As these drugs opened asthmatic airways and relieved symptoms, they did little to counteract the underlying disease. And so the inflamed tissues silently worsened. I compare this approach to prescribing a diabetic insulin *and* a pound of sugar cubes, or a heart patient medicine *and* deep-fat-fried foods. What is the point of giving a person drugs if you go on exposing them to the very factors that are causing their illness?

A new rash of studies shows that asthma deaths are indeed linked to asthma medications. The terrible irony is that the "cure" may actually be killing patients. Canadian researchers found that asthmatics who inhaled thirteen or more canisters of one asthma spray in a year (a bit more than one canister a month) increased their risk of dying *ninety* times. Those thirteen canisters were higher than the recommended limit, but many asthmatics become so dependent on sprays that they inhale much more than the recommended amount. Another report, just published last year in *The*

Lancet, one of England's most respected medical journals, found that frequent use *in normal doses* of some of these sprays ultimately worsens asthma.

The first crisis during my new age of drug use burst on me when I was sixteen. I had an asthma attack that just wouldn't go away. When I dragged myself to the doctor, he gave me prednisone, a powerful steroid. It was my first encounter with asthma's most potent and dangerous weapon. Prednisone is a drug that can, after long-term use, damage every organ system.

Yet it seemed like another miracle. I'll never forget how good I felt in just twenty-four hours. Not only could I breathe easily, I felt alert. My mood was elevated. I had a general sense of well-being.

For the next few years, whenever my lungs seemed to give out on me and the sprays didn't work, I'd just take prednisone for a few days. Short bursts of prednisone during acute attacks are actually the recommended method, but as I will explain in depth later, this approach should be a last resort, not a first line of defense.

Not until I entered medical school, where I worked and studied long hours, did a host of other problems begin to crop up. I began to pick up allergies of all kinds. I developed sensitivities to chalk, foam, dust, mold, pollen, wool, and foods. Above all, I was sensitive to formaldehyde, which happens to be one of the most toxic substances known to man. I frequently came into contact with it during my training in medicine, as organs are often embalmed in formaldehyde. My asthma worsened, as did my health generally.

Then came my first emergency room visit.

After my hospitalization, I was so ill my doctor placed me on seven drugs a day. I was taking huge doses of prednisone, doses beyond the limit for asthmatics, and included five other asthma drugs (terbutaline, theophylline,

Beclovent, Ventolin, and Humibid) along with Zantac, an anti-ulcer medicine (ulcers are a common side effect of prednisone). Every time I tried to go off the prednisone, I couldn't. I couldn't breathe without it.

If not used judiciously, most asthma medications can have disastrous and wide-ranging side effects, from skipped heartbeats, ulcers, mood swings, and mental clouding to bone loss, osteoporosis, and other even more threatening conditions, such as severe kidney damage and even death. I suffered many of these side effects. As the months passed, I became so weak and tired that sometimes I couldn't move, even get out of bed. I'd lie there conjuring a photo I'd seen in a medical report: a man lying dead in his bathroom with his asthma spray still in his hand. He'd died of heart failure linked to the overuse of his medications.

I could no longer sleep in my bedroom—the paint seemed to bother me—and one night my heart started skipping beats. Thinking that the all-ceramic bathroom might allow me to breathe, I curled up on the tiles and tried to sleep. My heart went on skipping beats through the night, and that morning I made an emergency trip to my cardiologist. He recommended yet another drug, Verapamil, to normalize my heartbeat.

Desperate, I asked my physician, Dr. Stuart Young, to request an emergency admission to the most famous respiratory institute in the country, the National Jewish Center for Allergy and Immunology. Their hospital has two hundred beds for asthmatics alone and draws emergency cases from all over the country. The institute, oddly enough, is located in Denver, at an altitude of over five thousand feet, which renders even those without respiratory problems short of breath.

I was astonished to find an entire institute set up just for the research and treatment of asthma, with intensive cross-disciplinary care, evaluating everything from the effects of Yellow Dye #5 to sulfites. I feel such a center can be invaluable for severe asthma, although a recent study reports that managed care companies are putting pressure on such clinics to justify their treatments. In 1990, asthma cost managed care $6.2 billion dollars. I believe a stay at a clinic such as National Jewish Center can be of crucial benefit.

At National Jewish, where I could rest and take stock of my rather desperate situation, my life took a new direction. For the first time, I realized that if I was ever going to get better, I'd have to take complete responsibility for my health. No doctor was going to save me but myself.

I had already begun to read some books about alternative treatments to asthma. I wasn't sure if it was simply desperation that was making me grab at straws. I asked the physicians at the center if they knew of any alternative treatments. They sent me to the psychiatrist. He asked me if I wanted to take a Rorschach test, which allows a psychiatrist to evaluate a patient based on his or her interpretations of inkblots.

"Doctor," I told him, "I just wanted information."

But the doctors began to lose patience with me when I kept on talking about alternative medicine.

I shut up. I was three thousand miles from home in the best asthma center in the country, and they were helping me. Some of their work, particularly on allergens and dyes, was brilliant. But I had turned a private corner. I had decided that I, a doctor, could no longer ask other doctors to save me. I had begun my break with convention—and embarked on a journey toward the rediscovery of health.

When I got home, I began to examine everything in my environment. I read every book and paper on alternative therapies that I could get my hands on, even if they were treatments in other parts of the world that were unaccepted here. I knew that, with my medical background, I was intelligent enough to distinguish between sloppy, flawed studies and those with genuine merit.

I was a detective on a mission. My first task was to create

a list of reactions I'd had to foods. Even when I was a toddler, I remembered eating a peanut and subsequently throwing up. And as I'd gotten older, I developed many other sensitivities.

Next, I took a close look at my environment. My home was decorated with shag carpet. Mold was growing underneath the carpet. Any wonder I'd been wheezing?

My office was located in a basement with cracked walls and no windows. It was part of a community clinic, and I felt committed to working there. Yet every time it rained, mold would flourish in those cracks. No wonder my sinuses hurt so badly so much of the time. The high doses of antibiotics I took to ward off my allergy-triggered sinus infections weren't doing me a lot of good, either. They were making me weaker and sicker and were completely missing the real problem.

I purified my diet. The food we eat can lead to asthma attacks because of allergies. In addition, preservatives and additives can cause allergies. Studies from the National Jewish Center for Allergy and Immunology directly link Food Dye #5 and sulfites to asthma for some sensitive individuals. The link between food allergies and asthma is too often overlooked. A recent report in the *New England Journal of Medicine* reported on fatal and near-fatal food reactions in children. Of the thirteen children studied, twelve suffered from asthma and food allergies. Six of these children died within a half-hour of eating the suspected food.

I then researched the mind-body link, hypnosis, biofeedback, and meditation. I now know we can harness the mind's incredible ability to calm itself and help heal the lungs. Scientists are discovering the profound link between mind and body: the interchangeable chemicals and receptors that our immune system and nervous system share. The two are able to signal each other directly, and there's no doubt that an alarm bell from the mind can trigger a cascade of inflammatory chemicals that help set off an asthma attack. On the other hand, techniques that help the mind alter the body's state can be so helpful that patients can often reduce their medications with these practices alone. Asthmatics can learn, through a step-by-step process, to relax themselves and significantly lessen the severity and frequency of attacks.

I began to read intensively in the area of mind-body medicine, and have continued to do so since that time. There are certain books that truly influenced me and helped widen my perspective. One of those was Dr. Bernie Siegel's *Love, Medicine and Miracles,* which offered inspiring accounts of healing from irreversible illnesses such as cancer, through a change in attitude, meditation, and visualization. Another important thinker is Dr. Deepak Chopra, who comes out of a tradition of Ayurvedic medicine, but whose broader message is the power of the mind to truly heal the body. Chopra maintains that each cell has consciousness, and that our thoughts can bring messages of healing to every cell in the body. A great innovator and thinker is Dr. Andrew Weil, whose recent bestseller, *Spontaneous Healing,* explained how to enhance your body's natural ability to maintain and heal itself—not just through good nutrition, but also through the mind's irrefutable impact on the body. Weil describes methods such as biofeedback and guided imagery, and describes some of his own healing experiences. Here is a quote from the wife of a patient who had nearly died from a brain tumor: "If I had believed the doctors all knew more than me, I would have accepted their pessimistic outlook and not kept pursuing the possibility of a cure . . . Harvey has been reborn . . . I've been reborn in the process too. Our adventure has inspired both of us to keep trying to heal the parts of ourselves that are not yet healed."

If, even in the darker moments of discomfort and despair over chronic illness, we can muster our faith and hope, and allow our minds to lead our bodies with the hope of being not just "cured" but reborn, we can go a long way toward influencing our health.

I learned about the importance of breathing, and I practiced breathing exercises. Like most asthmatics, I had never learned to breathe properly and fully. I learned how to use a peak flow meter, a device as necessary to the asthmatic as a driver's license is to the rest of us.

I researched the effects of vitamins, minerals, and antioxidants on chronic illness. There are almost no large-scale studies on the impact of vitamins and nutrition on asthma, a situation that must change. Studies cost tens of millions of dollars, and since you can't patent a vitamin, definitive studies will rarely be funded. Nonetheless, more and more research around the world has shown that vitamins are effective in helping delay or combat almost every known illness, from birth defects in children to heart disease and cancer. And now, studies on a wide range of vitamins and minerals show that certain key nutrients, including selenium and magnesium, tend to be low in asthmatics. As noted in the *Journal of the American Dietetic Association*, magnesium deficiency can contribute to lung problems. The *American Journal of Medicine* also supports the use of magnesium in asthma. I concluded that nutrients could make a difference, and so I supplemented my diet.

Most important, I examined my attitude. Until I'd been hospitalized, I'd tried to ignore and deny my asthma. I see patients like that all the time. One came in yesterday. She was feeling so much better on my program that she stopped coming and began to slip into her old lifestyle. She went to smoky bars, stopped watching her diet, stopped taking her vitamins, and stopped her breathing exercises. When she came back to me and we tested her lung capacity, her breathing ability had dropped to only 25 percent of the normal flow. If she hadn't come back to me then, she would have ended up in the hospital a few weeks later, pumped with intravenous drugs and steroids. Now she's back on my program, and she's fine.

Today, I know my lungs are a truly sensitive barometer of

toxins in my environment. Asthma is on the increase because, in part, our world is so toxic. Fifty thousand new chemicals have been released into the atmosphere since 1949, and we've only investigated a handful of them. I now respect my body's demand that I avoid as many of these chemicals and toxins as I can. If you are asthmatic and you want to get well, you can take nothing in your environment for granted. Once you structure your life with this in mind, it becomes natural and automatic. And the benefit is that priceless gift—health.

That is my story, and it can also be yours. You are the person who is ultimately responsible for taking the steps to ensure your health. You too can avail yourself of the wealth of good information available. The big difference between you and me, in fact, is that I am offering you all the knowledge it took me years of practice and research to assemble.

Today, I am off all seven drugs prescribed to me at the time of my hospitalization. I still take an occasional bronchodilating spray. My asthma is so improved that I can now work fourteen-hour days, host a weekly radio show, give frequent lectures, teach at a local university, and take breaks to run in Central Park or play tennis. I am directing studies on the effect of specific nutrients on cancer cell cultures with a grant from the Royal Academy of Medicine in Sweden, as well as their effect on asthma and on other chronic illnesses of our time.

I feel better than I have ever felt in my life. I'm writing this book because I know every asthmatic can lead a healthy, full, and active life.

In treating asthmatics, I've come to understand a lot about the stages of asthma. I've come to recognize the long-term stages of the condition. Having gone through the agony myself, I have absolute empathy for the asthmatic. When you can't walk half a foot because you can't breathe—that's no way to live.

A life on drugs is not the answer, either. Drugs can be lifesavers in an emergency, but over the long term, drugs didn't help me—nor have they truly helped the countless numbers of asthmatics who have gone on suffering or even died in recent years. If you're interested in drugs, there are many books that explain their benefits and side effects. That's not what this book is about. This book is your guide to a lifestyle revolution that will restore vitality and health—not just help you breathe.

In spite of years of suffering, I now consider myself fortunate in some respects to be asthmatic. Asthma forces me to avoid toxins and pollutants that end up contributing to cancer and other degenerative diseases later in life.

A forty-five-year-old patient of mine stopped by this week to say affectionately: "I feel so good I think I'm dreaming." Another patient, a twenty-one-year-old model whose career was stonewalled, was unable to breathe or leave the house. She was chronically fatigued and dependent on prednisone and asthma sprays. She suffered from frequent colds and flus. The final straw was when she had to turn down a modeling assignment in Europe: her face had gotten puffy from the prednisone. Today she is off her drugs and just appeared on the cover of a national magazine.

Just as inspiring are the children I treat. I remember my own childhood and how asthma limited it. If you can help an asthmatic child get well, you are preserving his or her lungs for a lifetime. One six-year-old I am now treating had been hospitalized twice this year. He suffered not only from asthma but from hyperactivity. On my program, he has now been off his medications for four months.

This book is unique because it offers a treatment program discovered by a medical doctor who recovered beyond all expectations from his own asthma. If you are one of the 25 million asthmatics alive today, read this book. You can be the next one to recover.

CHAPTER TWO

Getting to Know You

Until now, there has never been a comprehensive program for the treatment of asthma: a program that truly addresses every aspect of a patient's life. That's because most physicians look at asthma as a very specific condition of the lungs, and they treat it with medications targeted to symptoms.

I look at asthma as a complex puzzle that involves the truly intricate web of your body's immune and nervous systems. To me, asthma is the focal point for a larger problem. Proof of that is that I rarely find an asthmatic who simply has respiratory problems and feels great otherwise. Almost invariably asthmatics suffer from allergies, fatigue, back pain, frequent upper respiratory and sinus infections, and malaise.

Asthma is above all an inflammatory condition. Most doctors would agree on that point. However, we should also be asking: What regulates inflammation? Chronic inflammation is regulated in large part by the immune system, and the immune system is greatly influenced by the nervous system. That's why my program proceeds step-by-step, analyzing and treating every factor that might contribute to the asthmatic condition. It serves as an overall bridge between medication and natural therapy, with the goal of getting you healthy naturally.

I call my approach the Comprehensive Asthma Prevention program (CAP). As I mentioned in chapter 1, it is a program that addresses every possible trigger of asthma, from the way you breathe to the level of vitamins and minerals in your red and white blood cells to the toxins in your home and office. But the first part of my program is getting to know you—really getting to know you.

As a reader of this book, you are like a potential patient who has come to me to learn about your asthma, to understand the myriad factors that trigger it and to discover how you can vastly improve your health. All kinds of questions may be running through your mind: How can I prevent asthma? What are the latest studies about my condition? Are certain medications dangerous? What kind of changes go on in the lungs of a person with mild asthma? Can I exercise if I have asthma? What kind of exercise is best for me? Do children outgrow asthma, or is that a myth? Why are asthma sprays associated with so many deaths? Do allergies to molds make me vulnerable to asthma?

We can answer many of these questions. We live in a time that is truly remarkable for asthma research. Researchers have exciting insights into the cascade of chemical interactions that result in asthma. Science has made significant discoveries about neurotransmitters, receptors, and a special class of important inflammatory chemicals called interleukins. (Even now drug companies are working on medicines based on some of these discoveries.) We are learning that immune and other cells in our body may be malfunctioning even though blood tests come up normal.

Some forward-thinking physicians are taking the insights of this new line of research and raising preventive, holistic medicine to a far more sophisticated level. We are on the verge of utilizing an advanced class of tests—not just ordinary blood tests, but techniques that can truly help give you an accurate "fingerprint" impression of your level of health or illness. This new wave of medicine focuses on how well each organ and system in your body actually functions. It looks at what happens in your body before you show dramatic and overt symptoms like an asthma attack. The new approach to medicine examines just what is going on at the cellular level. After all, asthma (like any illness) occurs at a cellular level, and that is the level where you must begin to heal it.

I combine this exciting, informative battery of tests with traditional allergy and blood tests, so that I can direct a patient's recovery in a very specific fashion. I am like a detective who gathers information from every source: you, your history, symptoms, lifestyle, family's health, and a broad range of tests. As you read this book, consider it a guide to help you and your physician chart the same course of healing that a patient of mine would follow.

HOW ARE YOU?

When we meet, the first thing I do is a history and physical exam. In addition, I look for seven specific signs:

1. Are you breathing properly, using your diaphragmatic muscles to inhale, or are you using other muscles to help you breathe? Asthmatics often use their accessory muscles to breathe, lifting their shoulders as they inhale. This gives them a hunched look, which is especially obvious in people who have suffered from asthma for many years.

2. Are you able to complete your sentences? An asthmatic often has to take breaths while talking and is unable to actually complete a sentence without taking a short, wheezy breath.

3. Do you have a rapid pulse? A rapid pulse can be due to side effects from medications, anxiety, or simply

because asthmatics do not have enough oxygen in their systems.

4. Are you wheezing? Is the wheeze audible? Is it heavy and raspy, or light and mild? Wheezing indicates that you have mucus plugs blocking your airways.

5. Is there no wheeze at all? Sometimes this is a danger sign, as it can indicate that an asthmatic has lost the ability to draw in enough air.

6. Are you anxious? An asthmatic often feels anxiety, triggered by the inability to draw in air.

7. Do you suffer from abdominal, back, or sternum pain, or tenderness in the ribs? All these symptoms can indicate that you are using your chest muscles too heavily as you attempt to breathe, straining the muscles and resulting in a sensation of pain or tenderness around the ribcage. By checking these seven common indicators, I can gain a preliminary sense of how severe your asthma is. If you have any three out of these seven signs, you may have an acute, significant problem with asthma.

YOUR STORY

My next step is to ask to hear your story. Each human is unique, and so the disease called asthma manifests differently in every individual. Listen to a few different stories from my patients, and think of your own history as you read this. What turning points stand out in your own experience of asthma?

Michelle, a twenty-nine-year-old, suffered most of her life from severe allergic asthma. When she first entered my office, she told me her story:

My earliest memory of asthma was when I was six years old and went to the circus. I remember my dad dropping us off, I remember seeing the elephants, and the next thing I knew I could not breathe and I was doubled over.

I would get attacks every three or four months, mostly in reaction to animals. I would be fine, and then suddenly I couldn't breathe.

Later in my life, when I got to college I got really sick. Maybe it was the different trees there in the mountains, or the fact that the dorms had really dry radiator heat. All I know is I got really sick but I kept going to classes anyway.

One day I couldn't breathe at all. I went to the health clinic, the doctor gave me a shot, and it didn't help. He gave me another and nothing happened, and the next thing I knew, they put me in a wheelchair and were speeding me down these hospital corridors. I ended up in intensive care with all these people around me and monitors everywhere, and it seemed like they put me on every drug imaginable. I felt like I was hallucinating. After that, they prescribed inhalers, and for years, it seemed like I was dependent on them.

Seven years later, I had to be hospitalized again, and it was even worse. I felt like I was a number without a name, that they punched a computer and gave me a list of medications and sent me home without ever taking into consideration what was unique about me. And I said to myself, "There is no way I'm ever going to a hospital again. There's got to be something I can do. I don't want to be drugged up and put on a conveyer belt." Doctor, that's why I'm here.

Another patient, Rob, was a thirty-eight-year-old producer of television commercials whose asthma had begun when he was eight years old. When he came to see me, he was run down and suffered from toxic levels of medications, particularly theophylline.

I'm taking 900 milligrams of theophylline a day, and I'm afraid to go off it, Doctor. I'm afraid I won't be able to breathe without it. I'm feeling jittery and I can't sleep well, and my personality seems different than it was when I was younger. I feel more anxious and exhausted than I ever have and I can't exercise at all. I'm afraid to make plans, travel, or even be alone, because I never know how my asthma is going to be. I used to be the king of spontaneity, and now I'm hesitant to say yes to anything.

Mary, a forty-seven-year-old, developed asthma when she was forty-two. Until then, she had been fine.

I suffered from a few bouts of bronchitis one year, and they were really lingering, and one day I had this strange feeling, as if I couldn't breathe. I felt completely panicky, and that happened to me again and again over the next six months. I had about nine major attacks where I had to go to the emergency room, and one time I was housesitting and had to call a cab to go to the hospital by myself. When I was out of the hospital, they put me on high doses of drugs, and I started getting bad headaches and terrible insomnia. It seemed like all the energy I ever had just drained out of me, and I had to cut back my job to just a few days a week. I must admit I don't feel very hopeful. I've read so many things and heard so many promises, and nothing has really helped me. [Mary was able to stop taking theophylline within two months of her treatment in my office, and her energy and strength have come back.]

Each of these patients had a different story, and the onset of their asthma was distinctly different, although all shared the asthmatic's typical lament: "I am afraid to do anything. . . . I can't travel because of this. . . . I can't go to restaurants. . . . I can't even go over to my friend's house." (Some patients become so accustomed to a sedentary lifestyle that they have practically forgotten how enjoyable life used to be.)

For Michelle, allergies were a prime cause of asthma, and until those allergies were treated, we could not even begin to look at the other factors in her illness. In Rob's case, mild, lifelong asthma had been worsened by drugs that depleted his immune system, and until he was weaned off the drugs, he would continue to suffer fatigue and low immunity, which would only make him more vulnerable than ever to asthma attacks. For Mary, infections such as bronchitis damaged her lungs, setting her up for full-blown asthma. In her case, we had to immediately focus on boosting the immune system aggressively.

THE COMPREHENSIVE ASTHMA PREVENTION PROGRAM QUESTIONNAIRE

As you can see, each patient is a complex puzzle. For that reason, I like to give a special questionnaire in addition to the standard questionnaire you might fill out at any doctor's office. A standard questionnaire asks about your overall history and health, as well as your family's health. It inquires into major common illnesses, such as diabetes, heart disease, and cancer, and asks you to list past surgeries as well as medications you might be taking. But a standard questionnaire (along with standard blood tests) ignores entire areas of an asthmatic's life that may be prime causes of their condition. If you imagine a pie cut into twelve or fourteen different pieces, each of those pie pieces represents an area of your life that might be triggering your asthma. And within each piece of pie are specific factors and clues. They indicate to me just which allergy and blood tests I should recommend and what treatments I should emphasize.

My CAP questionnaire is unique because it is a directed questionnaire, designed specifically for asthmatics. It underscores many of the health hazards we are facing in the twentieth century, hazards often not associated with asthma. I ask about such seemingly far-flung information as the amount of animal fat in your diet or whether you work near a photocopy machine. Because I want you to participate actively in your own healing, I explain the theory behind my questions. This is what makes my program different and more effective.

I suggest you take time to fill out this questionnaire now and see just how many questions you answer 'yes' to. As you read this book, you will understand why I ask specific questions and what the answers may indicate. You can refer to your CAP questionnaire throughout this book. If your score is high in one or more particular areas, do not despair. I will show you how to improve your health. Once you have begun to locate the prime sources of your asthma, you can begin to take steps to improve it.

CAP QUESTIONNAIRE

Instructions: Answer the following questions. Except when otherwise indicated, score a single point for every "yes" answer, and zero for each "no" answer.

DRUGS

1. Asthma medications. Are you taking or have you taken in the past any of the following drugs (score half the designated points for a drug you are no longer taking):
   a. oral steroids? (5)
   b. inhaled steroids? (3)

    c. theophylline? (3)

    d. beta-agonist inhalers? (3)

    e. other daily asthma medications? (2 each) Please list dosage and frequency.

2. Allergy medications. Are you taking any medications, such as antihistamines, for allergies? (2) For sinus-related allergies? (2)

3. Hormones. Have you ever or are you now taking birth-control pills? (1)

4. Antibiotics. Have you ever or are you now taking antibiotics? (2) Please list antibiotics you have taken in the last five years. Did you take these antibiotics for upper-respiratory infections like bronchitis, pneumonia, and ear or sinus infections? (1 for each)

5. Do you use any other drugs frequently? (2 for each category)

    a. Antidepressants?

    b. Zantac?

    c. Blood pressure or cardiac medications, including beta blockers?

    d. Antifungal medications?

    e. Any other drugs? (1 each)

For all the above medications, please list the name of the medication and the dosage prescribed.

HOME

1. Do you feel better away from home? (1)

2. Do you notice symptoms

    a. in your bedroom? (1)

    b. in your bathroom? (1)

3. Is your mattress without an allergy-proof cover? (1) Do your pillows contain natural feathers or down? (1)

4. Is your bedroom carpeted? (1)

5. Do you use an electric blanket or electric heater? (1)

6. Do you notice symptoms after exposure to any of these (¼ point each): soaps, solvents, bleaches, ammonia, polishes, floor waxes, moth balls, varnish, hair spray, perfumes (including magazine strips), newsprint?

7. Has your home been recently renovated? Recently

painted? Recently carpeted? If so, is your carpet synthetic? Have you recently bought new furniture? (1 for each yes)
8. Do you feel worse after using vacuum cleaners? (1)
9. Is your home heated by forced air? (1)
10. Is a fireplace or wood-burning stove used? (1)
11. Does your home have a humidifier? (1/2)
12. Does your home have an air conditioner? (1/2)
13. Do you feel better when in your air-conditioned room? (1)
14. Do you or does anyone in your family have special hobbies that use potentially hazardous materials (such as glues or paints or cleaners and solvents)? (1)

OFFICE

1. Has your office been recently renovated? (1)
2. Do you work near a photocopy machine or laser printer? (1)
3. Is there adequate ventilation in your office? (1 for no)
4. Are your symptoms worse at work? (1)
5. Do you work with any hazardous materials, such as paints, solvents, cleaners, inks, dyes, glues? (1)
6. Do you feel better when in an air-conditioned office? (1)
7. Does anyone smoke in your office? (2)
8. Are ventilation systems used throughout the building? (1 for no)
9. Is your office heated by forced air? (1)

FOOD

1. Do you notice any of the following symptoms immediately after eating: fatigue, shortness of breath, wheezing, stuffy nose, runny nose, hives, itching, flushing, feeling hot, feeling cold? (1 for each)
2. Do you eat a varied diet with plenty of vegetables and fruits? (1 for no)
3. Do you eat a lot of "junk," refined, or fried food? (2) Please list the junk foods you eat.
4. Do you eat meat frequently? (2) Do you eat fatty rather than lean meat? (1)

5. Do you drink alcohol more than twice a week? (2) Occasionally? (1)
6. Do you crave certain foods or sweets? (1) Please list those foods.
7. Are you taking vitamins, minerals, and/or herbal supplements? (1 for no) Please list supplements, dosages, and brand names.

ALLERGIC POTENTIAL

1. If you have had allergy tests, were you positive for any of them? (1) Please specify the type of test: prick, scratch, or blood test.
2. Have you been tested for allergies in the last year? (Score 1 if your reaction was positive.) Please list the airborne allergens, molds, foods, and other substances to which you reacted.
3. Are you currently taking allergy injections? (1) For how long have you been taking them?
4. Do you suffer cluster headaches or migraines? (1)
5. Do damp rooms bother you? (1) Damp days? (1)
6. Do animals—for example, dogs or cats—bother you? (1)
7. Do you live in a heavily wooded area? (1)
8. Have you noticed a time of day (early morning, late afternoon) when your symptoms are worse? (1) Please note the time.
9. Do your symptoms flare in certain seasons or certain months? (1)

INTESTINAL DYSBIOSIS

1. Have you suffered side effects (such as diarrhea) from antibiotics? (1)
2. Do you suffer from frequent vaginal yeast or bacterial infections (women), or chronic irritation of the prostate gland (men)? (2)
3. Do you experience rectal itching? (1)
4. Do you experience itching after eating sweets? (1)
5. Do you have fungal infections around your nails? Ringworm? Jock itch? Athlete's foot? Thrush coating on your tongue? (1 for each yes)

6. Are you bothered by premenstrual symptoms? (1)
7. Do you experience bloating and gas after eating? (1)
8. Do you suffer from abdominal pain, diarrhea, or constipation? (2)
9. Do you suffer from
   a. joint pain, swelling, morning stiffness?
   b. irregular heartbeat, a sensation that your heart is going to beat itself out of your chest, or palpitations?
   c. aches in your muscles, painful aches after exercising, cramping?
   d. fatigue, mental cloudiness, irritability, shakiness?
   (Score ½ point for each yes answer above.)

IMMUNITY

1. Does anyone in your family—sibling, mother, father, grandparents, cousins—suffer from asthma? (1)
2. Have you ever been hospitalized for asthma? How frequently? (1 for each hospitalization)
3. How often have you suffered from pneumonia or bronchitis? (1 for each time)
4. Do you suffer from frequent colds and flu? (2)
5. Do you exercise at least three times a week? (1 for no)
6. Does physical exercise worsen your condition? (1)
7. Do you feel worse after sudden changes in temperature? (1)
8. Do you wake up at night? (1)
9. Do you wake up in the early morning (about 5 A.M.)? (1)
10. Do you wake up after a good night's sleep feeling tired or short of breath? (2)
11. Do you meditate or perform other relaxation techniques regularly? (1 for no)
12. Do you practice deep, diaphragmatic breathing? (1 for no)
13. Are you experiencing any difficulties in your life, such as a recent death in the family, loss of a loved one, divorce, or other stress? (1)

NUTRITION

1. Do you suffer from dry, rough skin, dry eyes, or night blindness? (This could indicate a deficiency of vitamin A.) (¼ for each)
2. Do you suffer from easy bruising, frequent infections, slow wound healing, bleeding gums, nosebleeds? (This could indicate a need for more vitamin C.) (¼ for each)
3. Do you suffer from vomiting, depression, headaches, nausea, constipation, fatigue, irritability, and lack of appetite? (This could indicate a vitamin B_1 deficiency.) (¼ for each)
4. Do you suffer from inflammation of the tongue, cracks at the corner of the mouth, and patches of dry, itchy skin? (This could indicate a vitamin B_6 deficiency.) (¼ for each)
5. Do you suffer from a sore tongue, weight loss, weakness, back pains? (This could indicate a need for vitamin B_{12}.) (¼ for each)
6. Do you suffer from weakness, headaches, sleeplessness, anemia, irritability? (This could indicate a deficiency of folic acid.) (¼ for each)
7. Do you suffer from muscle weakness, shortness of breath, fatigue, dizziness, tingling in the fingers and toes, anemia? (You may need more iron.) (¼ for each)
8. Do you suffer from a loss of appetite, loss of taste sensitivity, dull hair color, skin changes, and poor wound healing? (You may need more zinc.) (¼ for each)
9. Do you suffer from muscle cramps and spasms, fatigue, tension, irritability, loss of coordination? (These symptoms might indicate a need for magnesium.) (¼ for each)

Finally: Add up your sectional totals to get your overall score.

Well, you may be heaving a sigh of relief now that you have plowed through this long and perhaps seemingly unorthodox questionnaire. Many patients seem stunned by the range of topics dealt with, and they ask: "Is it possible that so many things actually affect my asthma?" It is indeed.

In sum, before I begin any treatment for a patient, I take a complete history, listen to their personal story, and administer a detailed CAP questionnaire. Then I have before me a veritable treasure of clues to just what is causing their asthma and where to begin focusing treatment.

Then comes the next step. I explain what an individual's score indicates. And then, based on my analysis of their score and their personal history, I recommend a series of both traditional and cutting-edge laboratory tests to give me a complete biochemical fingerprint of each individual. Then treatment can truly begin.

So if you were a bit mystified by the questions I asked, look at chapter 3 to learn about my underlying philosophy of asthma, and why and how the CAP questionnaire is a key to your return to health.

DOCTOR'S RECOMMENDATIONS FOR ACTION

1. Get a complete physical exam from your physician. Ask him to check for the seven most common signs of asthma.

2. Write a brief history of your experience with asthma, from your first episode up to the present time. Try to look for any common themes, such as allergies, seasonal episodes, environmental triggers, and so on.

3. Take the CAP questionnaire.

CHAPTER THREE

Putting the Puzzle Together

Pretend—once again—that you are in my office, this time for your second appointment. You've answered the CAP questionnaire and told me your own story. In turn, I've told you about some of the unique testing I offer to help puzzle out possible triggers for your asthma. In fact, I may have already ordered some tests and may have the results in your patient folder. Where do you stand now?

This is the time when we pause to analyze your case and map out the initial direction of your treatment program. First, we will go over your questionnaire together and look at your scores. Both your sectional scores and your total score are extremely important. Your overall score gives me an indication of how much you are suffering from your asthma on a day-to-day basis. Your sectional scores point to areas we must focus on. If you score high in any given section, we will pay special attention to that area and begin to treat it first.

Let's go, section by section, through the questionnaire and the meaning of the scores.

DRUGS

As you may have noticed, I take drugs seriously. I believe they should be prescribed judiciously and monitored closely. They can be lifesavers and can improve the quality of living, but they can also be abused. I believe medications can contribute to your illness if used too liberally, especially if they are not given in the context of a healing program.

First, medications can sometimes worsen your symptoms. Medications can have potent side effects, including palpitations, irritability, fatigue, headaches, and nervousness. Long-term effects of steroids, for instance, include osteoporosis, lowered immunity, and yeast infection. These side effects can exacerbate asthma and can be confused with the symptoms of asthma.

Drugs may also create a rebound effect, so that your condition is worse when you are not taking the medication. Further, they put continual extra stress on your liver, because they must be metabolized and detoxified. That extra stress can fatigue an asthmatic, whose entire body is already working overtime.

I am concerned about several different types of drugs: asthma and allergy medications, antibiotics, and hormones. The drugs you are taking can give me some important clues to your symptoms. For instance, you may be taking antibiotics for recurring bronchitis. Yet this may not be the ideal solution, since frequent upper-respiratory infections are a sign that allergies may be present. The allergies may be causing tissue to become inflamed and then become vulnerable to infections. Long term, antibiotics may not be a wise or effective solution. Studies show that when suspect foods are eliminated, recurring infections often clear up for good.

Hormones, in particular, are an important regulator in asthma, particularly the hormones secreted by the adrenal glands.

Antihistamines can leave you drowsy and fatigued, and they may not be beneficial to your overall health. A recent and alarming animal study found that certain commonly prescribed antihistamines potentiated the growth of malignant tumors in animals. However, long-term effects in humans are not known.

Look at your overall drug score:

- **Under 3 points.** You are most likely relying on drugs occasionally or for mild flare-ups but are probably not severely toxic from drugs. (There can, of course, be exceptions to this rule. For instance, an asthmatic taking only steroids might score only 4 but be suffering serious side effects from this potent medication.)
- **4–10 points.** You are relying too heavily on drugs to treat your symptoms. You are probably stressing your system and quite possibly suffering from side effects.
- **10 points or more.** We must focus on reducing your drug load immediately. You are suffering side effects and severely stressing your system.

Note: If you have been on steroids for over a year, I will probably suggest a bone density test to check for signs of osteoporosis. If you seem to be suffering side effects from theophylline, I will test for blood levels of the medication to be sure they are in the normal range.

HOME AND OFFICE

Your home environment should be an oasis where there are absolutely no allergens present, yet the opposite is true for most of my patients. Their homes contain needless environmental hazards, molds, dust, and other allergens. Carpet and bedding can be sources of dust mites, which cause allergies to dust, and vacuum cleaners may actually stir up settled dust and molds. Everything from shower curtains to synthetic fabrics and carpets to certain electrical devices can release formaldehyde gases, which may worsen allergies and asthma. Many common household cleaners and products give off toxins. Heating systems can blow molds, bacteria, and pet dander into the air. Humidifiers can harbor molds and bacteria, and if they overmoisturize the air, mold growth in the home may be stimulated. Air conditioners can also be a blessing and a curse, because they can sometimes harbor molds that grow rapidly in the condensed vapor when the machines are not being used, and are then released into the air when the air conditioners are turned on.

Your office can be a source of the same allergens and toxins as your home. Air-conditioning and heating systems may harbor molds and bacteria. Renovation using modern materials may expose you to countless chemicals, toxins, and gases that may worsen your asthma.

According to the recently published textbook *Chemical Sensitivity* (volume 1: *Principles and Mechanisms),* by Dr. William J. Rea, increasing numbers of Americans are experiencing a bewildering range of chronic complaints, many of which are due to sensitivity to toxins in the environment. Dr. Rea and his associates at the Environmental Health Center in Dallas, Texas, have treated more than twenty thousand such patients and have found that vitamins and minerals are depleted as the body attempts to detoxify substances. Most chemically sensitive patients have accumulated toxins in their bodies. Toxins tend to build up in cell membranes. Ironically, some individuals who work in toxic offices may actually feel worse on the weekends, when they go home and their bodies are able to begin to eliminate the toxins—causing symptoms of illness.

Look at your combined home and office scores:

- **Under 4 points.** You are probably not suffering in a significant way from toxic exposures in the home and/or office, unless there are individual exposures (a particular office that may have been renovated, or a particularly moldy bathroom, for instance) that are bothering you.
- **4–14 points.** You are definitely being exposed to toxins in the home and/or office but probably have not suffered serious immune damage from exposure. You still have a chance to clean up your act!
- **15 points or more.** Your exposure to toxins in the home and/or office is high and is harming your health. You need to address this situation immediately.

If your score in this section is moderate or high, I will recommend a thorough evaluation of your home and office (see chapter 9). I may test you for sensitivities to certain molds and will look at your overall IgE (Immunoglobulin E) score to determine how violently you are reacting to allergens and toxins. I may also recommend a hair analysis test to see if you are storing up toxic levels of heavy metals, or a caffeine clearance test to see how well your liver is detoxifying toxins (see chapter 4).

FOOD

Foods can have a dramatic impact on asthma in several different ways. First, you may be suffering from food allergies and sensitivities that keep inflammatory chemicals circulating in your body, thereby making the likelihood of an asthma attack greater. Second, certain foods have been demonstrated in studies to increase levels of inflammation in the body. Junk and fried foods and fatty meats can produce inflammatory by-products. Flax oil or fish oils can do just the opposite: they tend to reduce inflammation.

Those individuals who drink regularly are subject to liver toxicity, caused by excessive alcohol. This is particularly dangerous for asthmatics: their livers are already working overtime because their bodies produce a lot of toxins during asthma attacks.

Many of my patients crave sweets, which may indicate reactive hypoglycemia, food allergies, low blood sugar, or perhaps a deficiency in serotonin, a brain neurotransmitter. This condition can make you feel your asthma is worse, because symptoms include shakiness, panic, and weakness. These symptoms may be confused with asthmatic symptoms, setting off a vicious cycle.

Finally, my patients—although they often are already taking some vitamin and herbal supplements—are not usually targeting these supplements as specifically as I do as part of a complete program. I need to know exactly what you are taking, including the brand name. I am an ardent advocate of nutrients, but many vitamins and minerals may contain binders and fillers to which you may be sensitive or which may make them hard to digest. In addition, some herbal or natural products may contain compounds that are related to grasses and pollens that cause allergies.

Look at your overall score in the food section:

- **Under 4 points.** Your diet is basically good and is probably not harming your health or digestion.
- **4–7 points.** Your diet needs to be cleaned up, and you need to be evaluated for food allergies and hypoglycemia.
- **8 points or more.** You need to take an immediate and honest look at your diet and how it may be adversely impacting your health.

In general, if your score in this section is high, I will emphasize a radical shift in diet to healthy meals (see chapter 8) and will be sure to recommend a nutritional blood panel that assesses your levels of vitamins and minerals. If your diet seems low in mineral-rich foods, I may recommend red blood cell mineral tests, particularly for magnesium and zinc, two nutrients essential to an asthmatic's health.

ALLERGIES

Allergies are a key to asthma, as even mainstream, classically trained physicians admit, and allergies can change over time. The ever-popular allergy shots can sometimes take several years before a benefit is noted, so there are questions about whether improvement is due to a placebo effect or to simply outgrowing allergies. An indication of food allergy, for instance, might be a recurring headache; a frequent indication of mold allergy might be an inability to tolerate damp days or damp rooms, with symptoms of stuffiness, confusion, a feeling of mental cloudiness, sneezing, and wheezing. Allergies to grasses and trees are usually seasonal; morning allergies are often due to mold and pollution, and afternoon allergies are often related to pollens.

Look at your allergy score:

- **Under 3 points.** Your allergies are probably rather mild, and though we will test you for some allergies (suggested by your personal history), they do not need immediate focus.
- **5–9 points.** You suffer from moderate allergies, and they may be an important cause of asthma attacks. We will discuss your personal history and recommend testing based on clues in your own life.
- **10 points or more.** Allergies are a serious problem for you and need immediate focus.

In general, my first step is to test you for allergies. I will also recommend an overall IgE test. Then we can begin to address your allergies through desensitization, immune-boosting treatments, and avoidance of allergens whenever possible.

INTESTINAL DYSBIOSIS

You may be amazed to learn that the surface area of your intestinal tract is as big as a tennis court, and that within its coils reside 80 percent of your immune system. Digestion cannot be underestimated as a factor in any chronic illness, including asthma.

Bacterial and fungal overgrowth in the intestinal tract can lead to a host of problems, including a weakening of the immune system. The intestinal lining is part of the immune system, as you will learn later in this book. An overgrowth of pathogenic bacteria and yeasts is often caused by poor diet along with frequent use of antibiotics, which disrupt the normal balance of the intestinal flora. An overgrowth of "unfriendly" or harmful flora can impair your body's ability to produce digestive enzymes and stomach acid, which help to properly and completely digest food. Infection with the bacterium Helicobacter pylori, which has been linked to ulcers, has recently been linked to hay fever, sinusitis, and other allergies.

These harmful microbes can also release toxins, leading to an inflamed, permeable intestinal lining. This is known as "leaky gut" syndrome. A leaky gut allows inflammatory chemicals and undigested food molecules to pass into the bloodstream, causing inflammation in other parts of the body, such as the joints or the lungs.

Look at your dysbiosis score:

• **Under 4 points.** Your digestion is very probably adequate or good.

- **5–9 points.** You may have a problem with dysbiosis, or leaky gut syndrome, leading to allergies to food. I recommend a comprehensive stool analysis to determine the levels of healthy and pathogenic bacteria in your gut.
- **10 points or more.** This indicates a significant number of symptoms are related to your intestinal health. I recommend a comprehensive stool analysis and specific tests to determine if you are suffering from malabsorption syndrome.

What is a comprehensive digestive stool analysis? This test will examine the stool to determine how well you are digesting fats, proteins, and carbohydrates, how much fiber is in your diet, and whether you have an overgrowth of undesirable bacteria or yeasts. I may also recommend some tests to determine if you are suffering from malabsorption, or from intestinal permeability (known as leaky gut syndrome). In addition, I may test the ph level of your stool. Some individuals with food allergies suffer from subnormal levels of stomach acid, and supplementation improves their symptoms.

IMMUNITY

Immunity is influenced by both "nature" and "nurture"—by your genetic inheritance, or the capacities you were born with, and by your lifestyle, or how much you support your health through proper exercise, breathing, and nutrition. You can gain some clues to your genetic template by looking at your family history. Do allergies run in the family? Is there a history of certain conditions (such as asthma, heart disease, diabetes)?

Your current immune status can be assessed by looking at your ability to sleep properly, to exercise, to stay out of hospital emergency rooms, to avoid frequent infections, and to withstand seasonal changes in temperature.

In addition, mind and body are profoundly linked. A whole new field of research, called psychoneuroimmunology, has begun to look at the links between the mind ("psych"), the nervous system ("neuro"), and the immune system ("immuno"). Exciting new research shows a continuous feedback loop between mind and body. In particular, there is a direct link between emotion and flare-ups of any chronic illness, including asthma.

Look at your immunity score:

- **Under 4 points.** Your immunity is intact, even though you are under some stress. This is a good time for you to learn techniques for staying healthy and handling stress effectively over the long term.
- **4–9 points.** Your stress levels are high and may be adversely impacting your health and immunity. You need to begin a stress reduction program now.
- **10 points or more.** You are overloaded with stress and may even feel you are at the breaking point. You may not know it, but your body is using up valuable stores of stress hormones and nutrients, and your ability to recover from stress is significantly impaired. You can be tremendously helped by focusing on immune-boosting techniques and stress-reduction exercises described later in this book.

If you score high in this section, I may recommend several tests of your immune function. These include a test of your white blood cells—called T-cells—which can indicate underlying infection.

NUTRITION

Over time, subtle vitamin deficiencies can lead to immune depression, which only makes it harder for your body to heal itself after an asthma attack. In addition, studies and biopsies of asthmatic lungs have shown that certain nutrients are often deficient.

Look at your nutrition score:

- **Under 4 points.** Subtle deficiencies are most likely not a problem for you. Even so, asthmatics require extra nutrients to return their lungs to a healthy state. A proper regimen of nutrients and healthy oils is important for you.
- **4–6 points.** You may be suffering from subclinical nutrient deficiencies. A complete diagnostic nutritional workup is recommended.
- **7 points or more.** You are probably suffering from nutritional deficiencies that are severe enough to cause symptoms. A nutritional workup is recommended immediately.

If you are suffering from symptoms of vitamin and mineral deficiency, I will recommend a complete nutritional blood profile. We will focus immediately on boosting your immune system through healthy foods and nutrient supplementation (see chapter 7).

YOUR OVERALL CAP SCORE

I recently took the CAP questionnaire myself, though I answered the questions according to my state of illness at the time when my asthma was at its worst. That was a time when I was not only hospitalized, I nearly died.

My score was 57.

Theoretically, one could score well over 100 points on the questionnaire, but almost nobody does. These questions are specifically pinpointed to get at symptoms and triggers of asthma, and I feel that any score above 30 is very serious. Here is my basic breakdown for overall scores:

- **Under 7 points.** Your asthma is probably mild, although even at this level you may be suffering from uncomfortable symptoms, be taking too many drugs, and impairing your health over the long term.
- **7–20 points.** This is a moderate score indicating that there are definite triggers in your lifestyle and environment for your asthma, but that it is not yet out of control. You still have time to correct any initial damage!
- **20–30 points.** This score indicates that your asthma is a significant problem and a program such as CAP is recommended to prevent permanent damage to your lungs.
- **30 points or more.** Your asthma is serious! You need to follow a program like CAP with commitment to preserving your health and helping your body repair the damage done from this chronic illness.

WHAT CAN YOU DO?

You've answered the questionnaire, added up your points, and now have a better sense of just where you stand. This book provides a clear and detailed step by step approach to regaining your health. While you can implement many of its suggestions on your own, as with any illness, asthma requires the care and guidance of your physician, especially when medications and nutritional deficiencies are a factor.

Take a look at your section scores. If you scored high on allergic potential, pay special attention to the chapter on allergies, and ask your doctor to help you address that area of your life immediately. If you seem to be suffering from nutritional deficiencies, turn to the chapter on nutrition and read about the latest advances in nutritional information, and follow a general protocol for asthma. If you scored high in intestinal dysbiosis, you may want to ask for a stool test by a laboratory that specializes in intestinal dysbiosis, and you may want to pay special attention to the chapter that addresses this problem. Once you are aware of the "red-hot" areas of your life, you can make appropriate changes.

If your overall score was high, do not use it to create more stress for yourself! Remember, I myself was taking seven different medications and had my own brush with death in the hospital before my life began to change. Knowledge is power. Now that you know more about the possible causes of your asthma, you can begin to correct them.

You may like to do the questionnaire again in six months to see how you have progressed.

DOCTOR'S RECOMMENDATIONS FOR ACTION

1. Review your overall scores for each section of the CAP questionnaire—drugs, environment, food, allergy, intestinal dysbiosis, immunity, and nutrition. Make a note of any medium or high scores.

2. Pay special attention to the chapter or chapters dealing with an area where you scored moderately or extremely high.

CHAPTER FOUR

Your Unique Biochemical Fingerprint

Each patient has his or her own unique genetic and biochemical imprint. I am often amazed to find how subtle,
complex, and individual this imprint is. Like a spider's
silken web, woven differently each time, each person's biochemistry is unique. Each patient has a special combination
of hidden nutritional deficiencies, allergies, and sensitivities. Every patient also has unique healing capacities that,
when tapped, can help restore health.

Now is a time when science is rapidly advancing, and our
ability to understand our biology is breathtaking. We are
mapping the human gene, a feat only recently deemed
impossible, and we are beginning to understand how vitamins and nutrients are involved in the intricate biochemistry of health and illness. Major universities are performing
much of this research, and a whole new class of sophisticated, high-tech tests is developing. I utilize some of these
tests in my practice whenever I can. Once we have a detailed
picture of a patient's individual chemistry, the CAP program can begin in earnest.

Once you and I have talked and I have looked over your
questionnaire, the next step of my program begins. I will

schedule you for a battery of tests, based on the information and signs gleaned from your story.

Suppose, for instance, you are like Rachel, a twenty-two-year-old actress. Her history and questionnaire indicated that she suffered from allergies to animals, dust, and molds. She also appeared to be suffering from nutritional deficiencies of several B vitamins and magnesium, contributing to constant fatigue and a pale, sallow complexion. Another patient, Rick, scored poorly on questions about digestive difficulties. Digestive problems can be uniquely linked to asthma and allergies, as you will discover later in this book. I immediately scheduled allergy tests for Rachel, mold tests for her home, and a complete nutritional profile. For Rick, I immediately scheduled special tests to determine the level of inflammation in his intestinal wall.

In this chapter, I will explain all the tests I use, innovative new tests that get to the root of each patient's problem. These tests are selected carefully for each patient in order to minimize cost and save time. At first, you may be surprised at some of the tests, since they seem to have little or nothing to do with your lungs. As many physicians today are just beginning to understand, however, different organ systems in your body are profoundly linked to the health of your lungs, and your overall health as well.

In addition, I will explain low-tech ways you can help determine your own biochemical fingerprint in case you do not have access to a physician who will readily perform these tests. Tests can be expensive, especially some of the newer ones, which may not be covered by all insurance companies. In every case, I try to choose tests that are covered by insurance, and to be extremely selective, using only those tests that I deem essential.

Here is an overview of the tests, both traditional and new, that I use to get a picture of your biochemical fingerprint.

ALLERGY TESTS

Allergy testing is becoming increasingly important in the recovery of patients. The following is a brief overview.

Skin allergy tests. Many physicians will test for allergies by giving you scratch, intradermal, or prick tests on the skin. They are quite common and can be useful indicators of an allergy. In intradermal testing, a small amount of allergen is actually injected under the skin. Scratch tests are done with a scarifier, which is a device that scratches the skin, then a drop of the allergen is placed onto the scratch site. In prick or puncture tests, the allergen is already on an applicator that pricks the skin. In response to all of the above testing methods, allergies are generally indicated by a red weal, which varies in size and color intensity. This weal is then carefully measured to determine the level of sensitivity.

When another technique called serial dilution is used, increasingly stronger dilutions are injected under the skin—in other words, weaker and weaker doses—until the correct dose for neutralizing the reaction is determined. The correct dose seems to shut off the allergic response. Finally, there is a blood test called RAST testing which can also test for a wide range of allergies.

I utilize a variety of methods for testing, and my choice is always based on what is the best method for each individual patient.

Most patients complain that allergy testing is tedious and uncomfortable. It involves hours at a time, for many days or weeks. However, a new test makes allergy testing infinitely easier, faster, and more pleasant. Those of you who are accustomed to getting scratch-tested dozens of times will be amazed by this new skin test.

Called MultiTest, it is a panel that can test for eight allergens at once, by giving two rows of four equally spaced puncture marks. At each site, an exact amount of allergen is released, so that one can compare the resulting weals more accurately. This is far more efficient and rapid than traditional testing, where one must test substance by substance. Hundreds of potential allergens, from molds to foods to chemicals, are available to be tested by this method.

In general, I will test patients for eight to thirty different allergens. I choose these tests after looking over their personal history and questionnaire and determining what the likely allergens are.

Total IgE. I will then, fairly often, perform this highly informative test, which looks at how allergic your body is overall. *IgE* stands for Immunoglobulin E, and it is the primary allergic antibody formed by your immune system when you're exposed to an allergen. It occurs almost immediately, when the body mistakes the protein of a harmless substance (such as the saliva of dogs or cats) for the protein of a harmful invader. IgE molecules are released in a kind of waterfall cascade that sets off a chain reaction in your body, resulting in asthma and allergies.

A total IgE test is an instant indicator of just how allergic you are. IgE is an antibody that promotes many of the other inflammatory reactions in your body, and it does this by fitting onto the receptors of a cell called the mast cell, which releases a flood of histamine and sets off a cascade of complex chemicals that incite even more inflammation. In my experience, IgE is found in much higher levels in asthmatics than in other allergic individuals, and the higher your level of IgE, the more likely you are to have severe asthma, according to a 1992 study in the *New England Journal of Medicine.* An even newer test, the Phadiotop, tests for environmental allergens as a class. I will be evaluating this test soon.

A quick look at your IgE score, and I will have a good sense of how you are reacting today to irritants in your environment, from pollens to dogs and cats to dust. This test also tells me how severe your general condition is and how quickly or slowly I should take you off steroids or other medications (if you are on them). If your score is very high, I will be careful to wean you slowly from any medications that help dampen allergic reactions. A more moderate score, in turn, may mean that you will not be quite as dependent on the steroids, even if you are taking them. Your body has more of a "buffer" zone.

Other blood tests. On occasion, I also perform a few other special blood tests for allergies. One commonly used is the *IgE RAST (radio adsorbent spectophotometry)* for individual allergies such as mold, dust, or pollens. I find it useful for patients who have skin disorders, severe skin reactions, or severe or potentially fatal reactions to certain allergens. In such cases, it is far safer to draw blood and test the blood in the laboratory, even if it is not a perfect test.

A blood test for allergy that may be available soon is *cationic eosinophilia.* Eosinophils are rather amazing little cells that are part of the late stage of inflammation. Unfortunately, they are also often present in high quantities in allergies. When you have high levels of eosinophils in your blood, these cells can move almost instantly to a site of inflammation, creating further havoc. Studies have documented that eosinophils are involved in narrowing of the airways and tissue damage in the lungs. When asthmatic lungs are biopsied after death, there is always a great deal of eosinophil infiltration and resulting destruction of the mucosal lining. If your levels of eosinophils are high, your asthma most likely will be very active, and your lung tissue will be inflamed and damaged.

Blood levels of eosinophils are often measured in routine blood tests, but this test is completely different. This test will check for the number of active eosinophils that can instantly release their contents, causing tremendous inflammatory damage. I look forward to using it soon.

In sum, by looking at your total IgE and your allergy

tests, I get an instant and very accurate picture of just how allergic your system is and how active those allergies are right now. Remember, these levels can vary in each person according to the time of year. During the summer months, when pollen counts are often high, many asthmatic patients may have higher levels.

TESTS FOR VITAMINS AND MINERALS

As you will discover throughout this book and program, I cannot emphasize enough the importance of nutrition. How can your body begin to heal and to effectively neutralize allergens and toxins if it does not have the basic building blocks to mount a healthy response? I have found that anybody suffering from chronic illness and, therefore, chronic stress on the body has a higher than normal need for nutrients. Often, crucial nutrients are badly depleted by the day-in-day-out process of inflammation and illness. In fact, biopsies of asthmatic lungs reveal specific deficiencies in the tissues. Anybody who is allergic or asthmatic is in a constant state of battle with the environment, and they need to saturate their bodies with extra reserves of nutrients.

Most physicians do not test for levels of vitamins and minerals unless there are obvious deficiency symptoms that lead to clear, defined illness. For instance, a profound lack of vitamin C will lead to scurvy, and a severe deficiency of vitamin B_{12} can lead to deadly pernicious anemia.

Yet many people walking around with chronic conditions like asthma are also suffering from mild deficiencies. This can be particularly devastating if healing the chronic condition requires extra amounts of these nutrients. These tests are needed in individuals where questions exist as to their nutritional status.

Later in this book, in chapter 7, I will explain in detail the importance of specific nutrients, which can have a powerful impact on your health. Magnesium, for instance, is a proven muscle relaxant. It is a crucial nutrient for asthmatics.

Sodium, on the other hand, has been shown to worsen asthma. It causes tissues to retain water and swell. Other substances are also critical in asthma and may need to be tested for. Toxic metals like cadmium, mercury, or lead can inhibit the body's normal functioning, can block important enzymes in the body, and can displace necessary minerals from the cell. Cadmium, for example, blocks calcium and can have a wide range of harmful effects on cells throughout the body.

NutriSmart. A sophisticated laboratory test that I have designed, NutriSmart tells me if your body's levels of vitamins and minerals meet the government's recommended daily allowances. For instance, this test measures for vitamins A, C, B_1, B_6, B_{12}, folacin, iron, zinc, and magnesium. I also use nutritional testing from Bio Reference Laboratories.

Mineral panel. Some laboratories will perform a mineral panel (one I like to use is done by MetaMetrix Medical Laboratory, in Georgia). They will test for calcium, sodium, magnesium, and manganese in the blood, and for such potentially toxic minerals as arsenic, cadmium, lead, and mercury in the urine.

Hair analysis. Long scoffed at by most mainstream physicians, this technique has now been shown to be effective in detecting toxic metals. A recent article in *The Lancet,* the most prestigious medical journal in England, showed that hair analysis can be a useful indicator of mineral deficiency. Hair analysis is a very cheap and effective way to monitor toxic minerals in the body. However, these results need to be understood in their proper context. For instance, shampoos with zinc (such as Head and Shoulders) may give elevated zinc readings, and swimmers who frequent chlorinated pools show elevated copper levels in their hair.

Spectracell, Genox and Pantox Laboratories. Nutrition has become quite a respectable field of research of late, and one reason is the sophisticated testing now possible, which allows us to analyze exactly how the body's cells respond to vitamins and minerals. A recent front-page story in *Medical Tribune,* a newspaper widely read by physicians, spoke of the growing interest in nutritional and antioxidant testing as a wave of the future. These laboratories offer tests that give me a nutritional window through which I can "peer" into the health of your white blood cells, which are your body's first line of defense against infection.

These tests will tell me exactly which nutrients your body needs to be healthy. For even if blood levels on conventional tests are "normal," your actual requirements for specific nutrients may be high. You may have a genetic weakness in utilizing certain nutrients, or chronic illness and stress may be depleting your stores of nutrients quickly.

In one 1994 study reported by Luke Bucci, Ph.D., in *American Clinical Laboratory,* five randomly selected individuals were tested by one of these methods and given supplements to replenish deficient nutrients. A year later, they were tested. Seventy-nine percent of the tests that were initially abnormal had come into the normal range, and another 17 percent had moved toward the normal range.

I may recommend this test if you have been susceptible to many colds and upper-respiratory infections or are suffering from constant fatigue and low energy.

One test, called the Spectracell, works this way. White blood cells are cultured in a medium that provides the minimum amount of nutrients necessary for optimal function of the cells. Then particular nutrients are added one by one to the cell culture to see if the cells replicate faster or gain greater motility (ease of movement). If your cells respond to certain nutrients, that's a sign you need more of that nutrient.

In other words, this test measures the *endpoint* of nutrition—its effect on your lymphocytes. For instance, if your body needs more vitamin B_6, your lymphocytes will show a marked positive response when B_6 is added to a sample. These tests currently measure the functional status of up to nineteen different nutrients.

Nutritional analysis of red blood cells. Blood levels of nutrients are a useful indicator of your nutritional status, but they do not indicate how effectively your cells are "drinking" up levels of key nutrients. Regular tests only indicate how much of a vitamin or mineral is floating freely in your serum. Sometimes there is a big difference between levels of a nutrient in your blood cells, and the amount in your serum.

Red blood cell (RBC) magnesium. Magnesium is one of the most important nutrients on the planet where asthma is concerned, and yet despite its successful use in emergency rooms and hospitals since 1988, many asthmatics are completely unaware of its benefits. Intravenous magnesium has been used in hospitals to help treat severe attacks, and regular doses of magnesium can combat allergies, relax tight bronchial muscles, and increase energy. Magnesium is the crucial nutrient that helps relieve spasms in muscle cells. That is why, in asthmatics, you want to have active, high levels of magnesium. Magnesium is a regulator of cellular function in general, and a study published in *The Lancet* linked low magnesium levels to chronic fatigue syndrome.

Yet if magnesium cannot actually get into the cell, it won't work. A test for serum levels of magnesium—free-floating levels of the mineral in the blood itself—will tell you nothing about how the cell is functioning and how much magnesium it is managing to absorb.

Not surprisingly, I usually find low levels of red blood cell magnesium in my asthmatic patients. That indicates an immediate need for aggressive supplementation.

RBC zinc. Levels of zinc are terribly important in immunity, and individuals are far more susceptible to colds and flus when they are deficient in zinc. The elderly, in particular, have been found to be deficient in zinc. As with magnesium, serum levels are helpful, but they do not indicate how well the cell itself is absorbing zinc. I will test for RBC zinc if a patient reports many infections and colds. Some people have real difficulty absorbing zinc from their diet, even if they take supplements, and they need extra oral supplements, as well as intravenous supplementation to return levels to normal.

Other red blood cell tests are available, and I recommend them when necessary, for the same reason. Selenium, for instance, is important in immunity; it is a building block for many defenses in your body, and a powerful antioxidant used in dozens of enzymatic reactions in the body.

TESTS FOR ANTIOXIDANTS

Glutathione levels. One of the most potent antioxidants in the body is a substance known as glutathione. It is crucial in protecting the body from the destructive by-products of many chronic illnesses. Low levels are found in many inflammatory diseases such as asthma, and in cancer. And low levels of selenium, a mineral building block for glutathione, are commonly found in asthmatics. A study reported in *Thorax* found that low selenium levels increased the risk of asthma by as much as 5.8 times. Measuring blood levels allows me to accurately determine just how much glutathione or its precursors you may need as a supplement. Nonetheless, I recommend this test only rarely. That's because glutathione is so important that I recommend supplements that help boost its levels, no matter who the patient may be.

LOPS and T-BAR tests. These are the first generation of tests that measure actual free-radical damage in the body. Other, more sophisticated tests are likely to follow. I rarely recommend these tests because they can be expensive, but I mention them here because they are fascinating, can be useful, and indicate the direction in which medicine is going.

LOPS, or lipid peroxides, are rancid fatty acids in the blood. Performed by certain specialty labs, these tests will show me how many rancid fats are circulating in your blood. These fats are very closely linked to chronic inflammation and poor health. If levels of these fats are high, I will emphasize profound alterations in your diet that will help replace these rancid fats with healthy oils and fatty acids that help heal inflammation.

T-BARS (thiobarbituric reactive substances) are the breakdown products of these rancid fatty acids. These products have been linked to aging, illness, and heart disease.

If levels of LOPS and T-BARS are high, this indicates a high level of free-radical activity in your body. Though I will explain this in greater detail later in this book, free-radical damage is an important factor in asthma.

TESTS FOR DIGESTIVE PERMEABILITY: THE LEAKY GUT

Digestion? You may be pausing here and wondering if this test got into a book about asthma by mistake. Not at all! Did you know that most of your immune and lymph system is embedded in cells in the gut wall? Chronic illness and allergies are increasingly being linked to problems in the gut, including imbalances of disease-causing yeasts and bacteria (called dysbiosis), problems with fat and carbohydrate metabolism, and an inflamed gut wall that allows pathogens and toxins to leak into the bloodstream.

One primary way that problems in the gut occur is through poor digestion. When digestion is poor, nutrients from food are not absorbed. These undigested particles of food can affect the balance of bacteria in the gut. Harmful bacteria may feed off this food, creating bloating and gas and releasing toxins into your system. Certain bacteria, for instance, literally ferment sugar into alcohol or toxic aldehydes that are like ammonia. These toxic substances can create profound fatigue and can lower overall immunity. They will also cause the release of inflammatory chemicals, rendering you more allergic in general. I will explain this in clear, step-by-step detail in chapter 8.

There are several useful tests that can help indicate the state of your digestive system.

Comprehensive Stool Analysis. Laboratories such as Great Smokies Laboratory in North Carolina offer comprehensive stool analysis that detects how much undigested fat and fiber is in the stool, as well as the presence of pathogenic bacteria, yeasts, and parasites, all of which can cause chronic inflammation of the gut wall. Levels of beneficial bacteria, such as lactobacillus, are also tested.

Lactulose and mannitol test. This is a brand-new test that is not covered by insurance and is not yet in wide use. The test requires administering a solution of lactulose and mannitol to a patient who has fasted overnight, and then collecting urine. A person with a healthy gut will not absorb much lactulose and it will be excreted from the bowel unchanged. A person with an inflamed gut will absorb the lactulose, and it will appear in the urine. Mannitol, a sugar that is not metabolized by the body, is usually carried easily across the gut wall. If it is not quickly absorbed and later excreted in the urine, it means there may be a malabsorption problem in the gut.

Helicobacter pylori test. Amazing as it sounds, scientists now recognize that many duodenal and peptic ulcers and chronic gastritis are due to infection with this bacterium. (In fact, some cases of stomach cancer have been successfully treated by prescribing medications to kill this bacterium.) Because some asthmatics suffer from gastric reflux, where the contents of the stomach and stomach acids are regurgitated into the esophagus, causing chronic irritation, this test can be helpful in certain cases. I have seen several patients complaining of frequent cough and sore throat who were actually suffering from gastric reflux.

IMMUNE FUNCTION TESTS

Secretory IgA. This is an exciting test that can be help-ful to patients who suffer from frequent infections and colds. Secretory IgA (Immunoglobulin A) is an important indica-tor of immune function. If you are prone to getting sick, you may have low levels of available IgA, an immune anti-body that is a first line of defense against infection and is found only in the lining of mucous membranes, not in the blood. These antibodies have a broad antibacterial, antifun-gal, and antiviral activity. They are like the guards at the door, preventing enemy microbes from attaching to the mucous membranes and invading the internal system. When you suffer from many allergies, inflammatory chem-icals in the blood can use up much of your IgA. (IgA binds with the inflammatory chemicals, like a key fitting into a lock.)

This test can be performed by measuring the secretion of IgA in the saliva. This test, along with others, will indicate to me exactly where your immune system is weak and whether it should be boosted with specific supplements that raise levels of IgA.

PROCEDURES

Nasal laryngoscopy. Many patients suffer from sinus conditions that irritate the nasal and throat passages, setting the stage for lung inflammation. I may perform a test called nasal laryngoscopy, a relatively painless, in-office procedure in which a small tube is passed through the nose and enables me to detect nasal polyps, or inflamed tissue. I can also see fungal infections in the back of the throat and on the back of the tongue. Nasal polyps can be surgically removed, but they often recur, and I find that in 90 percent of patients, the polyp size can be painlessly reduced using a special aloe and saline solution, which I discuss in chapter 6.

"LOW-TECH" TESTING

Most of my patients will require only a few of all the tests I mentioned above. Here are several "low-tech" methods that I find very effective for determining your biochemical fingerprint:

1. You can use a food elimination diet to narrow your diet to a few, nonallergenic foods such as rice, vegetables, and a few fruits. You then test for food allergies by reintroducing foods into your diet, one by one. This is a time-consuming method, but it is the gold standard for food allergy. Many good books have been written about this method. One such book is *The Allergy Discovery Diet,* by John Postley, M.D.

2. A peak flow meter can be obtained from most pharmacies. This device, which I teach all my patients to use regularly, allows you to check your breathing before and after a meal, or before and after exposure to an allergen or toxin. This means that under the supervision of a physician, you can "challenge" yourself and find out if food allergies or something in your environment may be impairing your breathing ability. A peak flow meter can also be used before and after exercise, to determine if you have exercise-induced asthma.

3. In lieu of nutritional testing, you can sculpt your own nutritional program. I will explain the most common nutrient deficits suffered by asthmatics later in this book. I recommend high-quality vitamin supplements that contain no fillers or binders and that can be taken up to four times a day to generally boost levels of all nutrients. For some patients, I recommend specific, pure, high-grade vitamins and minerals in capsules, rather than a multivitamin, so I can be certain there are

no allergies to a particular formulation. Add a new vitamin or mineral each day. If you do not have any adverse reaction (or worsening of your asthma in general), move on to the next nutrient.

4. If you choose not to take tests for digestive permeability, take a clue from digestive disturbances such as bloating or irritable bowel. Add digestive enzymes and beneficial bacteria, such as acidophilus and bifidobacteria. Pay special attention to the chapter on nutrition, which details the effect of different diets, and emphasize antiinflammatory nutrients (e.g., fish oils) and healing nutrients (e.g., vitamin C and glutathione).

You have reached the end of phase one, or getting to know you. We will discuss the tests I recommend, and while we are testing you for allergies and/or waiting for the results of blood tests, we will begin to set up your individually tailored CAP program. It is an encompassing mind-body-spirit program, and therefore the next step is one where you pause to learn about asthma from a new perspective. Once you understand asthma in a new way, all the subsequent steps of the program will make sense to you.

DOCTOR'S RECOMMENDATIONS FOR ACTION

1. Recognize that each individual has a unique biochemical blueprint and that no case of asthma is exactly like any other case.

2. Adopt an attitude of hope and discovery. You are now working with me and your doctor to discover your own special biochemical needs and sensitivities.

3. Review your history, symptoms, and CAP question-

naire to determine, with your doctor, what special tests you might need.

4. Consider low-tech ways of detecting important information about your biochemistry. For instance, you can try an elimination diet as well as experimenting with different diets, and you can adopt a general asthma nutritional program.

CHAPTER FIVE

All About Asthma: A New Perspective

You've heard my story. You've answered the same kind of questionnaire that my patients fill out when they first come to my office. I've told you about the kind of testing I do, and suggested some low-tech ways that you can gain many of the benefits my patients obtain from sophisticated testing. Now what?

Now I take a moment to explain the basis of my approach to treating asthma, my special viewpoint on this condition. This point of view influences every treatment decision I make, every innovative and/or traditional healing modality that I adopt, and the way I assemble my CAP program. Once you understand the physical process of asthma the way I do, the actual steps of my program will make a great deal of sense.

Consider the fact that now more than ever is a truly remarkable time for asthma research, an era when many wonderful advances have been made in molecular biology and immunology. Today we know a great deal about asthma, and yet the asthmatic who has been yearning for this information has not found it easily available. It's hot off the presses of cutting-edge medical journals, but not much has been translated for the layperson.

Often my patients have read some of the other books available on treating asthma. Open any of the dozens of books on asthma and you'll find a chapter that explains, often in lavish detail, the physiology of breathing. Yet they rarely outline the essential truths of this condition and why it occurs.

To help you absorb what is, in many senses, a radical new perspective on asthma, I have organized this chapter according to the questions my patients most commonly ask me. These are questions about symptoms, treatments, and causes. Every answer reflects my new approach. When you finish this chapter you will, like my patients, have a changed understanding of this condition—and a new resolve that is grounded in insight.

The two most common questions my patients ask me—questions both simple and profoundly important—are: "What is asthma?" and "Why do I have it?" Doctors have been attempting to answer those questions ever since the ancient Greeks coined the word transliterated as *asthma,* which means "panting."

Q. What is asthma?
A. Before I explain what is going on in your body during an asthma attack, let me tell you a little bit about normal, healthy breathing. Your lungs are an exquisitely refined instrument that draws in air in precise amounts carefully regulated by your body's nervous system. Usually you do not even notice you are breathing, although your rate of inhalation and exhalation changes throughout the day to respond to your changing needs for oxygen—whether you are running on the beach, walking up and down stairs, or hunched in front of your computer spreadsheets.

Like your beating heart or your stomach as it digests food, your lungs function automatically. In fact, your respiratory system is aerodynamically designed so that breathing is as efficient as possible. First, air passes swiftly and easily in through your nasal passages, where it is warmed, humidified, and cleaned by tiny hairs. Then it moves swiftly down your windpipe to the branches of your bronchial tubes, which, because they are narrow, actually increase the speed at which the air moves. Then the air is distributed into your lungs (see fig. A, p. 70), where millions of evenly distributed air sacs called alveoli function like tiny factories (see fig. B), expanding and contracting as they absorb air and siphon out oxygen for your bloodstream, letting you exhale the waste product, carbon dioxide (see fig. C).

When this process goes awry during an asthma attack, it often begins with an allergen or irritant such as a virus, bacteria, fungus, or other toxin. The body responds by activating a vigorous inflammatory cell reaction to fight the "invader." Inflammatory cells go by odd-sounding names like eosinophils, mast cells, lymphocytes, basophils, neutrophils, and macrophages. These cells respond to the call to arms by releasing a cascade of toxic chemical weapons intended to kill the invader. Unfortunately, toxic proteins and peroxides destroy not only the enemy but also some of the tissue lining of the lung, where the body fears the invader may be hiding. When the damage reaches this level, new connective tissue is formed (much like a scar that repairs a wound), and over time, this process of damage and repair can lead to permanent scarring in the lining of the lungs. Even mild asthma has been proven to cause such changes, especially thickening and hardening in the lining of the lungs.

In response to this battle between the body and its invaders, the tissue lining the respiratory passages becomes swollen and air does not move as swiftly. Mucus is formed, to help protect the raw and irritated tissue, but mucus blocks airways and impairs the ability of the lungs to absorb oxygen. Irritated nerves send signals to the muscles surrounding the bronchial tubes, which tighten in spasm, making it harder to breathe. The result is the typical symptoms of asthma: wheezing, shortness of breath, coughing, phlegm, and chest tightness.

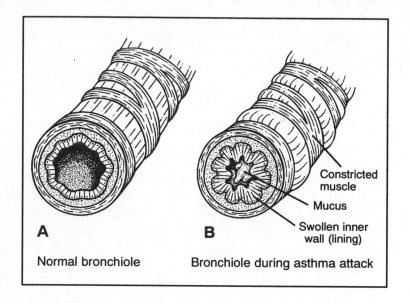

A
Normal bronchiole

B
Bronchiole during asthma attack

Constricted muscle
Mucus
Swollen inner wall (lining)

That is the first answer to your question. I would like to answer your question again, in a different way.

For a long time, asthma was defined as a *reversible airway disease.* Defining a disease is far different from describing it, but in essence this term means that during an attack, the airways become temporarily constricted and tight. That view of asthma paved the way for a generation of drugs that did one thing very well: they opened the airways. At the time, little attention was paid to the role of inflammation, now understood to be a hallmark of asthma.

Since that first definition, doctors have refined and rethought asthma. For a time, they classified the condition as either "intrinsic" (arising from internal causes) or "extrinsic" (arising from external causes). People with extrinsic asthma were understood to be allergic individuals who reacted to specific substances in the environment. The other asthmatics were a more mysterious and enigmatic group, and the cause of their asthma was said to be unknown.

Yet we now understand that asthma is far too complex to be divided into two simple groups. Many cases of intrinsic asthma may simply have been due to causes we didn't recognize, such as toxins in the workplace (from asbestos to formaldehyde to any other man-made substance). In addition, many allergies or sensitivities are not obvious and yet may contribute to asthma. Doctors will debate endlessly about the true nature and definition of allergy, but it's the patient's response that counts.

Modern-day descriptions of asthma have become far more technical and descriptive, and yet sometimes they seem like a medical version of "The Emperor's New Clothes." Consider this one: "chronic desquamating eosinophilic bronchitis," a term from the Mayo Clinic. That basically means there is extensive inflammation inside the lung with considerable debris clogging up the airways. This line of thinking is current and sees inflammation as the basic theme of asthma. That's why, today, steroids and antiinflammatory drugs are the major defense against asthma among many physicians.

I think they're still missing the point. Drugs should not be the centerpiece of asthma treatment. Countering inflammation with drugs alone will not help asthmatics reverse their illness. In fact, many of my patients already realize this when they come to me, and they are anxious about the prospect of drugs.

Q. How can you look at asthma as other than an inflammatory condition? Aren't the doctors right?

A. As I have said, they're right—but, I believe, only up to a point. I look at asthma from an entirely different point of view—a vantage point that is remarkably simple and yet guides me in every single treatment I offer. I think of the condition in terms of *free-radical damage and work.*

Free-Radical Damage. You may have heard a lot about free radicals, which I will explain in detail later. They are the by-products of combustion in the body: highly reactive, highly charged particles that need to be neutralized by the body or they will cause damage to your cells and genes. Free radicals are generated in great amounts during inflammation. The more free radicals that are generated, the harder the body has to work to clean them up. A study in the *American Journal of Clinical Nutrition* found that dietary antioxidants, which quench free-radical damage, can influence asthma. Vitamin C in particular was found to be extremely important in the lung. The study concluded that vitamin C may protect against free-radical damage.

Work. On the most basic level, the lungs work to give the body its most vital element: oxygen. Oxygen is the essence of life, the one necessity, the fuel for every combustion in the body. The need for oxygen—and the role of oxygen combustion in illness—is what makes asthma so distinctly different from other chronic diseases. Moment by moment, asthmatics must work harder to get oxygen to each cell, drawing air past clogged, narrow airways and struggling with each breath. At work, at home, walking, talking, even while sleeping, asthmatics are working overtime to draw precious oxygen into the body. Even in the deepest sleep, many asthmatics are still struggling to breathe. (In fact, asthma is often worse at night, and many sufferers of nocturnal asthma are wakened by the inability to breathe.)

I believe it's that day-in-day-out, year-in-year-out load of extra work that depletes asthmatics of vital energy, nutrients, and resilience. That may be why so many asthmatics are chronically exhausted and susceptible to frequent infections. Even more important, an asthmatic never knows when the body is going to be assaulted by a toxin that may precipitate an attack. The asthmatic, unlike those suffering from most other chronic illnesses, must always be prepared for a sudden assault.

Q. Can you explain to me exactly what that "work" involves?

A. First of all, it involves the mere act of breathing. Breathing is no simple affair. It requires work from a whole interlocking system of muscles and chemical messengers. Just the taking in and expelling of air is incredibly complicated. First the muscles of the nostrils contract, then the vertebral column extends, the muscles in the neck contract, the first rib moves upward, the internal diaphragm muscles contract and move the ribs downward, and the stomach muscles contract. In the lungs themselves, fluid is continually being suctioned into the capillaries from the space between the layers lining the lungs, and as oxygen combines with red blood cells, the brain sends out constant updates on the levels of oxygen in the blood. The respiratory centers in the brain never rest.

In asthma, where the lungs are inflamed and airways constricted, the brilliant aerodynamics of the respiratory system is profoundly altered. For instance, normally the nose warms, purifies, and humidifies air, so that by the time it reaches the lungs it is 98 percent saturated with moisture. If (as is often the case) mucus is plugging inflamed nasal passages, the asthmatic breathes through his or her mouth. The air is no longer conditioned and cleaned. It enters the lungs as dry, dusty, cool air. Second, as it flows into the lungs it encounters uneven, swollen, inflamed surfaces. That means it flows far less efficiently, with much less speed and pressure. In some asthmatics, the airway resistance can be as much as twenty-five times greater than normal.

Your bronchial muscles, your lungs, and the 300 million tiny balloons in the lungs—the alveoli, which draw in oxygen and expel carbon dioxide—have to work far harder. The lungs compensate by overinflating, trying to draw in more

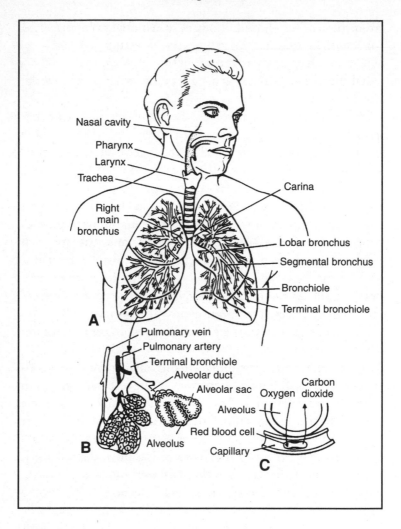

oxygen, and that stresses the muscles in the chest wall. Because oxygen levels may drop, the brain's respiratory centers have to work harder to monitor changes. If the body receives less oxygen, the function of every cell in the body is impaired.

It's impressive how efficiently many asthmatics perform

that monumental load of work, making sure that the body receives its elixir of oxygen. I've seen asthma sufferers who have lost half of their lung function and yet maintain normal blood levels of oxygen.

Yet that monumental effort can itself lead to damaged health and even death.

Q. Okay, your idea about work makes sense to me. But how can such a simple idea create a whole new approach to treating asthma?

A. Good question, and within the answer lies a key to the whole mystery of asthma. This condition is one of chronic inflammation, and so it generates more work for the body— the work of mopping up inflammatory chemicals and healing inflamed tissue.

During inflammation, huge amounts of free radicals are released. As the *American Journal of Respiratory and Critical Care Medicine* noted in June of 1995, allergic reactions in the lung lead to an influx of inflammatory cells. Free radicals are the by-products of energy reactions in the body, and they are highly reactive, highly charged particles that can damage cells. Free radicals are one of the most important concepts in disease, and free-radical quenchers may soon occupy as important a niche in medicine as antibiotics once did.

If we can combat free-radical damage—and the body uses huge amounts of energy working to do just that—we may be able to reverse, halt, or ameliorate many of our devastating chronic illnesses. In fact, the latest theory of AIDS and the ability of the HIV virus to trigger such a vast panorama of disease states now rests with free-radical damage: scientists at the National Institutes of Health have discovered that the virus blocks our body's normal defenses against free radicals. It may be free-radical damage that destroys immune cells and is one cause of AIDS. In fact, it may be free radicals that damage genes and lead to cancer, free radicals that damage tissue and lead to arthritis, free radicals that—once they have begun their damaging spiral—cause most chronic illnesses to steadily worsen.

When we consider asthma, free radicals are especially important, because free-radical damage occurs in the lungs, where oxygen is taken in. That means that every cell in the body is affected. I am always conscious of the fact that it's not just our lungs that breathe. Very few people think about the fact that each cell breathes and has a respiratory system of its own. The respiratory center in the cell is called the mitochondrion, and in this center, a complex chemical process takes place. Can you see now how asthma creates work, not just in terms of breathing but in terms of energy production in the cell itself?

Q. Yes, but it all sounds so complex. It's so far removed from my real life, where I wake up in the morning and I can't breathe. How can you take this theory and make it work for me?

A. We can actually move from theory to practice. We know a lot about how to fight free-radical damage and how cells breathe and function, and we are learning more every year. This is where I take a major departure in my approach to asthma. Drugs can be helpful, but they often work by suppressing the symptoms of inflammation. Inflammation is a specific reaction to an irritant or an allergen, and inflammation begets inflammation. It does this in large part because the by-products of inflammation are free radicals that damage tissue, causing further inflammation. Some drugs suppress inflammation without giving the body the extra boost it needs to repair itself. Other drugs, such as beta-agonists, ignore inflammation entirely.

I believe the best way to treat inflammation is by giving nutrients that slow down the inflammatory reaction and give the body all the resources it needs to repair tissue. In particular, I emphasize nutrients that help combat free radicals, help repair inflamed and damaged tissue, and give the body extra reserves of energy so that it can function well in spite of asthma. And I am no longer alone in this view. New studies find that supplementing selenium, which helps the body combat free-radical damage, actually improves asthma. One 1993 study in *Asthma* gave patients selenium for fourteen weeks and found significant improvement. Then, once the inflammatory reaction is slowed, I can focus on asthma treatments that ease the body's work, treatments that emphasize powerful breathing and strengthening exercises, relaxation exercises, purification of the environment, super nutrition, and specific free-radical quenchers.

As one example of how the concepts of work, free radicals, and cellular respiration can guide asthma treatment, let's look at magnesium, which, in high doses, relaxes smooth muscle. In fact, intravenous magnesium can reverse a severe asthma attack. A 1989 report in *Annals of Emergency Medicine* found that a seventy-two-year-old man whose lungs were failing after a severe asthma attack rapidly improved after intravenous magnesium, and was spared being put on a ventilator.

During an attack, the muscles surrounding the bronchial tubes are constricted, and when muscle cells contract, they do so because calcium has flooded into the cells and magnesium has drained out. Calcium and magnesium always work together in that way, a biochemical teeter-totter.

Calcium and magnesium have special significance in asthma. Without calcium, no muscle movement will occur, and that means no breathing. Too much or too little calcium will cause muscle spasms. In addition, excess calcium stimulates the allergic cell known as the mast cell, which bursts and releases inflammatory chemicals. Magnesium can reverse these problems naturally, most likely by displacing calcium in the cell.

Many studies prove magnesium's benefit; a study of seventeen asthmatic patients found that intravenous infusion of magnesium sulfate significantly decreased bronchial "hyperreactivity," or twitchiness, and substantially increased the ability of asthmatics to expel air (as measured by a peak flow meter). Another study found that during asthma attacks, magnesium levels in the blood dropped while histamine rose.

Magnesium can keep muscles from going into spasm. Thus, magnesium allows the patient to breathe easier. Ultimately, the work load decreases.

Here's another example. Antioxidants and free-radical quenchers can help clean up the debris from damaged, inflamed cells by assisting the body's own enzymes and by binding with and neutralizing the harmful by-products of inflammation. Thus, they are like cleanup crews that greatly ease the work of the body. Some of the most potent antioxidants available are vitamin C, zinc, N-acetylcysteine (an amino acid), beta-carotene, and some relative newcomers such as taurine, melatonin, and specific, highly active bioflavonoids. A May 1995 study in the *American Journal of Respiratory and Critical Care Medicine* found that diet may affect antioxidant levels and impact on airway inflammation. Simply put, women whose diets were high in vitamins C and E were less likely to suffer from asthma.

Fish oils are one of the most effective, natural antiinflammatory substances available to us, without the side effects of drugs like cortisone. Fish oils, like many other oils, work as a natural lubricant that allows cells to function more smoothly. Even more important, they actually are absorbed into the cell itself and continue working on a twenty-four-hour basis.

Each layer of a cell is lined with a fatty membrane, and many oils we consume are incorporated into that membrane. I suspect that by using an antiinflammatory oil that is absorbed into this membrane, we can help reverse inflammation naturally. Studies show that taking fish oils for ten weeks reduces inflammatory cells in the body, though it may take as long as six months to a year to see a substantial improvement in symptoms. (It takes the body time to repair damage that has built up over years!)

Q. But don't steroids block inflammation? I feel much better when I take steroids during a bad attack, and it sounds a lot easier than changing my whole lifestyle.

A. It's important to realize that you are changing your lifestyle in order to regain health. In the long run, you will have a far richer, more vital life, even if it takes more effort now.

It's easy to pop a pill. And, yes, steroids block inflammation, but they work on the very outer layer of the cell, where there are receptors for chemical messages. They profoundly alter the messages to those receptors, and I do find them beneficial for acute episodes and emergencies, where the doctor's prime objective is to get a patient breathing again.

Over the long term, however, steroids do not ease the body's workload. They actually deplete your body's stores of nutrients, including potassium, magnesium (which, as I mentioned, is very important in asthma), and calcium. Imagine wringing a sponge dry. That's what steroids do when used for long periods of time, and that's why they have such devastating long-term consequences, from osteoporosis to immune depression.

I recently treated a brilliant oncologist, a cancer specialist, who suffered from asthma and had been taking steroids for the past year. He had an overwhelmingly busy schedule. He felt chronically exhausted and sick and was ready to take a different approach to his condition. I tested his functional nutritional status with a NutriSmart test and was shocked to find that his nutrient levels were lower than AIDS patients I have treated. The steroids, combined with a poor diet and little sleep, had simply leached his body of most of his nutrient reserves.

The truth is that drugs often increase work, because they don't treat the cause, and yet at the same time often cause side effects. Drugs demand extra work of the liver and kidneys, which metabolize and excrete medication. That's why they must be used judiciously.

As you follow each phase of my program, you will begin to see how beautifully my treatments all work together—to reduce work!

Q. Why do you call asthma an immune disorder?

A. The key to asthma lies with the immune system. In active asthma, the immune system is ringing alarms all the way around the block—and ringing them overtime. An inflammatory avalanche has begun, and it seems to gather up everything in its path. It's as if the body has called out all its cops, and they are a bit punch-drunk with battle—on red alert for any possible invaders. Every newcomer is suspect. That's what's happening when you become oversensitive to your environment.

How does that happen? First, you must understand that the immune system is made of many types of cells that range freely throughout the body. Compare the immune system to a nomadic warrior tribe. Whenever an immune cell encounters an enemy—whether it's a cell that has turned cancerous, a microbe that can cause infection, or a man-made toxin—it calls in its soldiers to capture, kill, and dispose of the invader. However, in killing invaders, the immune system releases destructive forces that can damage the body itself. Other safekeepers of the immune system must turn off the alarm bells and clean up the damage.

In certain instances, those warrior forces seem to veer out of control, destroying innocent cells. That's what happens in many conditions like arthritis, colitis, or even asthma. In fact, it is now believed that many chronic viruses—such as those in the herpes family, or the Epstein-Barr virus, which commonly causes mononucleosis—may somehow upset the immune system permanently. Perhaps the constant presence of these viruses keeps part of the immune system on perpetual red alert. This dysregulation, or immune dysfunction, as it is called, can actually be measured. Laboratory tests have shown that in such cases the ratio of T-8 cells (known as T-helpers) to T-4 cells (known as T-suppressors) is reversed. There are too many T-8s in circulation, leading to constant inflammation.

Q. All this talk of T-8s and T-4s has confused me. I'd like to understand how the immune system fights an invader.

A. If you understand how the immune system fights a microbe or virus, you will begin to understand how it goes awry in asthma and in allergies. That will help you understand the basis of many of my treatments.

Here, very simply put, is how the immune system works when it encounters an enemy, which could be a virus, bacteria, or fungus—anything it regards as a threat. First, the invaders enter the body and are noticed by the body's frontline defenders, the macrophages. These cells are like Pac-Men whose mission in life is to gobble up foreign invaders. They begin to eat the invaders and then post little chemical "flags" that are like a warning. Those flags shout the enemy's "name."

The helper T-cell speeds by. It's the commander-in-chief of the immune system. It takes note of the enemy name on the macrophages and immediately begins to multiply, rushing to the spleen and the lymph nodes, where it orders other cells to fight the invasion. The killer T-cells heed the command and hightail it on a hunt for "infected" macrophages, killing them with a squirt of deadly hydrogen peroxide. Each time a T-cell kills a macrophage, the cell bursts and dies, spilling out its contents. Those contents will need to be cleaned up and carried away.

At the same time, the helper T-cell wakes up the B-cell. The B-cell produces chemical weapons called antibodies. These antibodies rush to the site of infection or invasion, where they tag the enemy for attack by other cells (like the killer T-cell).

As these cells do their jobs, they stimulate and release many chemicals that cause inflammation. Inflammation brings fresh blood to the area. The red-hot activity of inflammation is an indication that the body is attacking the invader.

Finally, the suppressor T-cells come along. Suppressor cells prevent the immune response from spiraling out of control. When they sense that the battle is being won, they slow down the body's artillery. Yet they leave memory T- and B-cells in the blood and the lymph system, ready to attack instantly if the invader should show up again.

Q. Since asthma is a problem of the immune system, is that why I get so many colds and bronchial infections?

A. In a sense, yes. In fact, some cases of asthma may initially be triggered by an infection of the lungs—perhaps due to a virus that stays in the lung tissue even after the acute infection is gone. (Other viruses, such as chicken pox, are known to incorporate themselves into our cells and stay there for life.) It is known as respiratory syncytial virus. For children in particular, this can have long-term harmful consequences, because damage occurs to the lungs while they are still growing, and remains for life. This virus usually attacks children before the age of two, and its presence may keep inflammatory immune cells circulating at higher levels than normal, leading to sensitivities to many other substances.

In fact, infection and allergy may be far more closely related than we now know. If, for example, the lining of the nose is chronically inflamed, sinus drainage can cause irritation all the way down the respiratory tract. That's one reason a common cold can soon flare into serious bronchitis, triggering the kind of asthma attack that ends in hospitalization.

So many more lingering colds and cases of chronic bronchitis are caused by allergies than we realize, and one indication of an infection triggered by an allergy is that it recurs with a certain pattern. Asthma patients often get colds in the winter. I believe unclean heating and ventilation systems in many homes and apartments may be a cause. They harbor bacteria and molds, which become airborne when vents are opened or heating systems turned on, and disturb the immune systems of sensitive individuals. Moisturizing and cleansing the air with humidifiers and air purifiers can eliminate allergic colds completely. (I explain this further in chapter 9.)

Q. Why does asthma often get worse over time?

A. Asthma and allergies seem to spread and worsen when inflammatory cells become "trigger-happy." Once inflammation is chronic, these cells are in constant circulation and can go off at the least sign of trouble. If too many soldiers, such as the macrophages, are out and about, they may become trigger-happy. In fact, we now know that mild and severe asthma look very similar in the lung: the inflammatory changes are not markedly different. That means that those with mild asthma may actually be at risk for a severe attack.

Q. What role does allergy play in asthma?

A. Allergies contribute greatly to asthma, and these allergies include not only sensitivities to pollens and dust mites but also to molds, foods, and chemicals. A landmark study in the *New England Journal of Medicine* found that of thirteen children who died of fatal food reactions, twelve suffered from asthma. Dr. Michael Kaliner, chief of the allergy division of the National Institutes of Health, has pointed out that allergy is the most common underlying cause of asthma.

New evidence shows that the prevalence of asthma is closely linked to an immune-globulin that is used to measure the intensity of allergies. This compound, known as

IgE, is present in high levels in the blood when an individual is highly allergic.

Scientists are studying other compounds that seem to be present in greater quantities during allergic reactions. One of the most interesting chemical mediators are the kinins. Bradykinins, for instance, are found to stimulate mucus production and other inflammatory chemicals, and they are present in the inflamed tissue of allergic persons.

I consider the treatment of allergies a mainstay of my program. I know simply because I suffered so badly from allergies myself, and they stressed my entire system. Even when allergies do not cause wheezing, they may be contributing to asthma. In my case, my sensitivities to foods are so specific that when I was at National Jewish Center's hospital in Denver, I could identify a "hidden" food by my reaction: tomatoes made me tired, wheat made me itchy, nuts made my lip swell. My asthma improved dramatically and immediately when I began to avoid all foods to which I had sensitivities.

Q. I get asthma flare-ups whenever I'm near a dog. I've noticed that when I go to my brother's house for the holidays and spend time around his two German shepherds, my asthma gets progressively worse each day. And I usually feel lousy for the next month. Why is that?

A. This is an excellent question, because it targets one of the most important aspects of asthma. Asthma attacks have more than a single stage.

Every asthma attack includes both an early- and late-phase reaction. The early phase is the initial attack, characterized by an acute reaction. It occurs within minutes of encountering an offending agent. That means as soon as you reach down to pet Spot, your brother's dog, you will start wheezing and sneezing. These are hallmark signs of inflammation and constriction, and they are primarily the result of the famous mast cell bursting. The mast cell is a key regulator of inflammation.

Once that mast cell bursts, it send signals to bring in other inflammatory cells. They are responsible for what is known as the late phase. This phase, which takes a few hours to develop, contains a whole cavalcade of immune and inflammatory cells. This double attack may be the body's version of dropping air bombs and then following up with ground troops.

Physicians now recognize that the late phase plays a crucial role in severe asthma. During the late phase, inflammatory chemicals are released that cause sustained constriction of the bronchial tubes and continued congestion. In any case, the late phase can persist long after the offending agent has been removed. These agents sensitize your lung tissues, so that your lungs will respond even more quickly and violently to an allergen. That's why your asthma steadily worsens when you're constantly around an offending agent.

Once this cycle is under way, the body is primed to attack irritants and substances the very moment they come into contact with the lungs. When asthmatics are continually living in the presence of toxins and allergens, there is little relief for damaged tissue. Inflammation stresses and depletes the body, creates more damage that is countered with further inflammation, and exhausts more nutrients in trying to clean up that inflammation. The cycle keeps doubling back on itself.

Q. Let's say I decide to try your program, because it makes sense to me and I'm willing to try something new. But what if my doctor disagrees with your approach?

A. This question brings up one of the most important aspects of your new path to health: your current doctor. Most of you who are reading this book are already seeing a physician who is treating your asthma. You may feel uncertain about breaking out in a new direction, and you may wonder whether "unorthodox" treatments are valid. Above all, you may be afraid to confront your doctor about the possibility of a change or of combining his or her treatment programs with mine.

Don't be discouraged. Partnership between patient and doctor is the new approach among forward-thinking physicians, who are willing to work with their patients to help create health.

That doesn't mean that you should play conductor to an orchestra of different physicians. You do need one doctor who knows the uniquely individual nature of your case and directs your care. On the other hand, physicians and patients can work together to educate each other.

Just last week I had a patient come to me and announce: "I want you to know you're the only doctor I'm seeing."

My response was: "That's fine, but it's not necessary. Next week I'm going to a conference on asthma and I'm going to spend three days sitting and listening to other physicians. Would I sit and listen to them if I thought I knew everything? Doctors learn from other doctors."

If your doctor is resistant to any treatment program but his or her own, I recommend that you encourage that professional to sit down and openly discuss options with you. This is particularly important if you feel attached to this individual. Inform your doctor that you are going to maintain contact with him or her while you attempt new therapies. Remind your physician that even if he or she feels unsure about the efficacy of these therapies, they may work for you. You are a statistic of 100 percent. If a new treatment helps you, it's 100 percent successful.

You may also wish to present your doctor with studies indicating the efficacy of certain treatments. You may even want to give him or her this book.

Occasionally, seeking out innovative treatments can lead to an outburst of anger on your physician's part. One patient of mine went back to her doctor after I'd given her a highly effective treatment with intravenous magnesium. He said to her: "Why are you throwing out your money on alternative treatments? That magnesium is just going to come out in your urine an hour later. Don't waste your hard-earned money!"

She was quick with a retort: "You've sent me for CAT scans, blood tests, and all kinds of procedures, and this is the first time I ever heard you mention anything about saving me money. Not only is this making me feel better, but I am functioning better and my peak-flow-meter scores are higher. And I have read studies to support it. I'd like to sit down and show you these studies and discuss it with you calmly."

If your doctor is adamantly opposed to any other treatment method but his own, it may be wise to seek out a new primary-care physician. In the appendix at the end of this book, I list organizations that can help you locate forward-thinking asthma specialists.

Hopefully, more and more doctors and patients will soon know about new treatment methods. I believe there is a paradigm shift going on in medicine in general—and in asthma in particular—a shift toward prevention of disease through immune enhancement. You, who are reading this book, are at the forefront of that change.

Q. Okay, you're making sense. But sometimes in the middle of the night when I can't breathe, I just wonder, Why do I have asthma in the first place? It's so frustrating.

A. This question is a bit like Pandora's box—it leads to a thousand other important questions about asthma. So I usually begin by answering it indirectly.

I want you to look around. Because if you do, you'll notice that you're not alone. The rates of asthma, chronic bronchitis, emphysema, and respiratory illness are soaring. All these conditions involve chronic inflammation of the airway tissue.

At least 15 percent of Americans also have a closely related condition, called allergic rhinitis, which involves inflammation of the nasal passages.

In sum, far too many Americans are suffering from some sort of respiratory illness, whether it affects the nose, the bronchial tubes, the lungs themselves, or all three.

So what is happening? Does a healthy, clean environment lead to an epidemic of respiratory disease? Of course not. Is it possible that asthma, a relatively unknown disease a hundred years ago, could suddenly appear out of nowhere, for no good reason? Highly doubtful!

Do we have a modern epidemic of pollution? Yes! Do too many of us eat a high-fat, high-sugar diet that is far from what nature intended to support healthy human life? Absolutely. Are we living in a society that dispenses drugs too freely? I believe so. Is this a world of high stress and frantic lifestyles that leave little room—literally!—to breathe? What do you think?

Couldn't asthma be an early-warning system—one that sets off an alarm in the presence of toxins? If we heed this alarm, I believe we can prevent years of damage to our health.

Asthma is one way your body—especially your lungs—tells you about the world you are living in. Is that world a healthy one?

Think of asthma as a mystery that you are now about to unravel, a mystery with clues scattered in many areas of your life. Let me show you how to listen to your body and your life, clean up your inner and outer environment, and ensure balanced good health.

DOCTOR'S RECOMMENDATIONS
FOR ACTION

1. Recognize that knowledge is power. It's important to understand the underlying causes of asthma and just what happens during an asthma attack. Then you can truly begin to change your health.

2. Begin to understand that asthma is more than a reversible airway disease. It is a condition that is the direct result of free radicals and an overstressed, overworked immune system.

3. Know that this book will teach you many ways to prevent and heal free-radical damage, particularly through very specific nutritional supplements targeted to known deficiencies that asthmatics suffer from.

4. Recognize that asthma attacks are not as simple as they sometimes seem. All asthma attacks involve an early- and late-phase reaction. Both phases need to be treated.

5. Try to enlist the help of your physican in adopting the CAP program. If your physician is resistant to discussion or is adamantly opposed to your trying some of the protocols discussed in this book, you may want to seek out another doctor to oversee your care.

CHAPTER SIX

Toward a Drug-Free Life

Often a new patient has come into my office and said, "I'm doing exactly what my doctor told me to do. I'm taking all my medications and I'm still miserable." Sometimes they will open a backpack or a purse and pour out a veritable pharmacy of inhalers and pills. Then they will look up innocently and ask: "What's wrong with me, Doctor?"

What's wrong? Too much medication, not enough medication, the wrong kind of medication, and most likely taken at the wrong time.

Medications, when properly used, are an invaluable tool. They can serve as a bridge to a healthier life. But too many asthma patients today are overmedicated and undertreated, or they are inadequately treated. They can make a dramatic improvement in their health by reducing their medication in the context of a program like CAP—a program that eliminates lifestyle triggers of asthma and bolsters the entire body with a rich lode of nutrients.

Because drugs are so potent, however, *no asthmatics should simply lessen their prescribed drugs on their own. This is one aspect of my program that absolutely must—without exception—be conducted under a physician's supervision.* You can read this book and make many of the changes in the CAP program on your own or with the care and help of a cooperative physician, but you risk serious health problems if you do not taper drug dosages under a doctor's strict supervision.

Most asthmatics are surprised to learn that they can start to taper off drugs they may have been using their entire lives, and that within weeks or months, they may be taking little or no medication at all. My contention is that although medication may be helpful and even necessary to save lives in some situations, you cannot get well while you are heavily drugged with powerful substances twenty-four hours a day.

My goal for each of my patients is simple and clear: to lead as healthy a life as possible while relying on the least amount of medication necessary. Ninety-five percent of my patients have reduced their medications significantly within the first six weeks of treatment. About 60 percent have cut them by at least half. Eight out of ten patients report a significant improvement in their general health soon after reducing their medication, and within three to six months 70 percent need to resort to medications only occasionally, if at all. Less than 10 percent take longer than six months to reduce their medications.

In this chapter, I will explain each class of drug and the different forms it comes in (and the different names it is called by). I will tell you which drugs are most popular and why; common and uncommon side effects (something your own doctor may not have told you); what indications make particular drugs appropriate; and what time of day to take them. Timing makes a big difference in the effectiveness of medication, particularly for asthma, which is regulated by hormones in the body, such as cortisone. (These hormones fluctuate in specific cycles each day, called circadian rhythms.)

As you read ahead, you will be learning facts about asthma medications that many physicians themselves do not know. One of the big tragedies in asthma is that this extraordinarily complex and potentially life-threatening disease, although it has reached epidemic proportions, does not have its own specialty or formalized training programs. I recently interviewed Dr. Stuart Young, chief of the Section on Allergy at Mt. Sinai Hospital in New York, about just this subject. "Residents are coming out of their training programs with virtually no understanding of allergies and only some understanding of asthma," he lamented. "There is an urgent need to train primary-care doctors about asthma."

Right now there are many different drugs offered for asthma, and new ones have been introduced as recently as this past year (salmeterol, for instance, a long-lasting beta-blocker spray). Even an experienced physician can be overwhelmed. Prescription drugs are not inherently bad, but the way they are sometimes prescribed in the specialty of asthma is wrong—often because physicians are not properly trained and have misconceptions about the real causes of asthma. Drugs are serious weapons, and they need to be used during times of genuine attack.

In case you think I am overzealous about the perils of drugs, let me remind you of the soaring rate of hospitalizations and deaths in this country from asthma—over 6.5 million visits to the hospital a year. We are literally pouring potent drugs and sprays down asthmatics' throats and telling huge numbers of otherwise healthy people that they will have to take exorbitantly expensive prescription drugs every day for the rest of their lives. Many of them are children. In this country between 1972 and 1985, prescriptions for asthma drugs tripled.

With a problem this massive, you would think a clear and rational treatment program would be in place, as it is for conditions like diabetes and heart disease. Yet, this has not happened. Read the following mind-boggling statement from one of our most prestigious medical publications, the *Journal of the American Medical Association,* which, in 1990, concluded: "There have been no long-term, randomized clinical trials to determine what constitutes optimal therapy in [asthma]." Here we have a major disease that is crippling our health care system, and we don't know what causes it, what drugs work best for it, and who should get those drugs.

Even more alarming is the fact that every decade we discard our latest "miracle" drugs because of their significant drawbacks. When I look back through the last few decades of medical articles, I'm amazed to find how often doctors keep revising their approach. I keep finding statements that emphasize changes in drug management: "Theophylline is not usually prescribed as a first-line drug in asthma management today." "Today, steroids are used only when bronchodilators have not relieved symptoms." "Now it is well recognized that excessive use of bronchodilators may result in more serious and long-lasting attacks." Which drug will be the next to fall from favor—and for good reason?

The fact is, we have not even done the most basic demographic studies of asthma, studies to show us which drugs work best in which populations. Perhaps children respond better to a certain class of drugs, while the elderly are more responsive to another set of medications. We have no real nuggets of information.

But here's what we do know: 7 million people suffered with asthma in 1980. Over 10 million suffered in 1990. In the 1980s alone, there was a 54 percent increase in the number of women who died from asthma, and a 23 percent rise in male mortality. Incredibly, our only answer so far has been more drugs. An article in a recent issue of the journal *Chest* noted that patients with severe attacks should not take more bronchodilating drugs because in a bad attack "the need for more bronchodilator is in fact a dire warning of the immediate need for another kind of treatment: oral steroids or hospital rescue." Hospital rescue, by the way, means intravenous steroids and theophylline—in large doses pumped straight into the bloodstream.

During an acute crisis, there is no wise choice but to get treated immediately, but once the crisis has passed, it's time to reevaluate. One patient of mine, Jane, came to me with very refractory, hard-to-treat asthma. Biweekly intravenous infusions of vitamins and magnesium proved so beneficial to her that her symptoms cleared up. She began to skip her treatments, and within a few months her symptoms returned. In Jane's case, her nutritional needs for certain nutrients are so high that she needs ongoing maintenance treatments in order to function effectively. Though this is not a cure, it is certainly far healthier for the body than a lifelong regimen of potent medications.

Keep these facts in mind as you read on and find out what the common asthma drugs are and how they work.

STEROIDS

Steroids are the most potent and most dangerous of all asthma medications available. Given in an emergency, they save lives. Given over time, they can irreversibly damage health.

I begin with steroids because they have become the treatment of choice today. There has been a change in the understanding of asthma. As I have already discussed, doctors once focused on airway constriction in asthma. Today, researchers understand that inflammation is the underlying cause of the disease. The answer that is often given is steroids, in one of three forms: intravenous (given in the hospital), oral (taken by mouth), and as oral sprays.

In fact, I fear this new era of steroids will only lead us down another dark alley. The truth is, doctors have known since the 1960s that asthma involved inflammation. Steroids have been an effective and potentially perilous treatment for just as long. Yet suddenly, everyone in the field of asthma and allergy is talking as if there were a chasm between our old understanding and our new understanding of asthma, and they apparently believe this new understanding will bring the disease under control. Why is nobody asking, "What is causing the inflammation?"

Take one of my patients, a forty-two-year-old photographer named Susan, who had been on oral steroids (prednisone), along with other medications, for a year. On her first visit, she brought me pictures of herself before she had gone on steroids. The woman who looked at me out of those photos was pretty, slender, and smiling. The woman in my office had a swollen face, puffy eyes, thin hair, and a hunched appearance. The steroids had literally disfigured her. (Anyone who has used high levels of steroids for over a year knows exactly what I mean.)

She was addicted to her steroids; unable to survive on less than 10 milligrams of the drug a day without suffering severe asthma attacks and bouts of fatigue. Yet she was experiencing some of the worst side effects: not just changes in her appearance, but early signs of osteoporosis, and mood swings that were putting great stress on her marriage.

In Susan's case, I started her on CAP while I weaned her off her oral prednisone. After about five weeks, I had reduced her steroids enough to start her on oral sprays, while continuing to reduce the oral dose. It took Susan ten weeks to wean herself completely off oral steroids and another four weeks to get off steroid sprays. Her appearance soon changed dramatically for the better: she looked healthy and attractive once again.

What Are Steroids?

Produced naturally in the body, steroids are hormones made by the outer layers of the adrenal glands. Steroids affect everything from the way we metabolize sugars and fats to the health of our immune system, and of course, they regulate inflammation.

Steroids were hailed as the miracle drug of the twentieth century soon after they were first synthesized in the laboratory. Their effect was shocking and dramatic, almost magically "curing" many devastating, intractable illnesses, from the agony of severe arthritis to chronic asthma.

Side Effects of Steroids

The miracle, however, carried a terrible price: as time wore on, the side effects of steroids kept mounting. Steroids, taken long-term, irreversibly harm, destroy, or disrupt virtually every organ in the body. Steroids force nutrients out of the cell at a much faster rate than normal, causing individuals to lose huge amounts of minerals that help maintain normal cell functioning. Numerous electrolyte and nutritional imbalances develop, and it takes the body time to repair them. Side effects include immune depression, poor wound healing, thinning of the skin, heart and lung damage, weight gain, high blood pressure, thinning of the bones (osteoporosis), joint pain, stomach bleeding, changes in fat metabolism, severe acne, extra hair growth (especially on the face in females), stunted growth in children, cataracts, mood disorders (including psychosis), suppression of the adrenal glands, leaching of precious minerals like potassium, calcium, and magnesium, and swelling of the face and ankles, giving steroid users a characteristic and freakish "balloon" appearance.

And this has now, once again, become the drug of choice?

Steroids powerfully suppress the adrenal glands. The brain responds to the artificially high blood levels of steroids by shutting down the natural production of the hormones, and if a patient continues taking the drugs over a period of months or years, the adrenal glands can actually wither away because they are not being used.

Trying to taper off steroids slowly is an absolute necessity—and often quite difficult, as symptoms can flare up as soon as the drug is reduced. It takes time for the adrenal glands to recover their function, and sometimes they simply fail completely, a dreaded complication called Cushing's syndrome.

A patient recently came to my office with the look of Cushing's syndrome. He walked in and sat down, and I knew before asking a single question that he had been taking high doses of steroids for a long time: he was moonfaced and humpbacked, with puffy eyes. The rest of his body was slender.

We have no clear idea just when steroids start to damage us. No one knows at what doses bone thinning or adrenal suppression occur. The current thinking is that most of the side effects of steroids occur at doses greater than 5 milligrams a day, since our bodies produce about that amount every day.

Some doctors maintain that "short-term" and "low-dose" steroid therapies do not cause significant side effects. I wish this were always true, but studies have shown that even a few days of steroids can suppress adrenal function temporarily. Adrenal suppression probably varies with each individual; some of us are far more sensitive than others.

Even inhaled steroids can cause damage. Many doctors recommend inhaled steroids because their doses are significantly lower than systemic steroids and because there is a common belief that inhaled steroids are not absorbed into the system in large amounts.

There is no doubt that inhaled steroids are a major improvement over the sledgehammer of oral steroids, and inhaled steroids used in the recommended dosages are generally safe. For instance, 1 milligram a day of inhaled steroids can control symptoms as well as up to 35 milligrams a day of oral steroids.

Inhaled steroids are, in fact, potent and can indeed have

damaging effects. We simply do not know what the effect might be in a child or adult who takes these sprays day in and day out. Inhaled steroids have been shown to have the major side effects typical of all steroids, including adrenal suppression, bone thinning, cataract formation, glaucoma, and a whole litany of unwelcome conditions.

Another routinely overlooked side effect of steroid sprays is fungal overgrowth in the mouth, called thrush, which can lead to persistent sore throats and difficulty swallowing. This may be mistaken for and treated as a strep throat. This means the sore throat, improperly treated, will remain persistent, since antibiotics actually perpetuate this condition.

Harry, a thirty-seven-year-old medical researcher for a news network, was suffering from asthma and came to me because of his ongoing sore throat. I knew that his constant sore throat could be due to gastric reflux, sinus drainage, complications from allergies, viral infection, or a yeast infection from his steroid sprays. I asked if he rinsed his mouth after spraying, and he said no. In addition, because he disliked the taste of his spray, AeroBid, he always ate candy afterward.

A laryngoscopy exam revealed white plaques at the back of his throat and tongue. A culture was positive for candida albicans, and we treated him with a powdered antifungal medicine, nystatin. He took it four times a day, after each dosage of AeroBid. The nystatin was dissolved in water, and Harry then swished it around in his mouth, gargled, and finally swallowed it to get the full effect. In addition, he cut sugar and candy out of his diet to avoid stimulating yeast growth. His sore throats cleared up.

If asthmatics with thrush take course after course of antibiotics for bronchitis and other infections, they are setting themselves up for a chronic yeast infection throughout the gastrointestinal tract and, in women, in the vaginal tract.

When Should You Take Steroids?

Are there times when steroids are appropriate?

Absolutely.

Prednisone is a drug that can rescue a patient in an emergency situation. In the hospital, in particular, intravenous steroids have snatched many an asthmatic from the jaws of death. Steroids can also help *prevent* potentially fatal attacks. Consider Bob, a patient who came in to see me recently and who had been wheezing for many years. He had relied solely on Ventolin, a beta-agonist marketed in spray form. His lung capacity was severely reduced and his respiratory muscles greatly weakened. In his case, an inhaled steroid for a few weeks helped reduce chronic inflammation that had gone completely untreated. Later I added osteopathic treatments, a manipulative therapy that adjusts the spine and helps balance nerve impulses to various parts of the body and has been shown to help asthma. It can be particularly beneficial for lung capacity, and these treatments along with breathing exercises brought his lung capacity back to normal.

Another patient of mine, Mary, was a seventy-year-old with chronic asthma. Shortly after she first came to see me, she came down with a bad winter flu. In an elderly patient, that situation can be dangerous and lead to a severe attack and hospitalization. I prescribed a short course of steroids for seven days, starting with 20 milligrams a day.

On the other hand, consider Johnny, a four-year-old child who, every time he was admitted to the hospital for an asthma attack, was administered an injection of steroids and sent home with a prescription for prednisone.

When a doctor and parents make a decision to put a child on steroids, they may have made a decision to alter that child's life forever. Immune suppression, shortened stature, thinning bones—these may be a lifelong legacy of early, prolonged steroid use.

A far better approach would be to say, "What might be triggering Johnny's asthma?" When I asked this question, I found out that his parents had just bought a new house and laid new carpeting down throughout. An environmental evaluation of their home revealed many toxins and allergens—from the formaldehyde gases and dust from the carpeting, to the molds and bacteria being circulated in the air by a heating system with dirty vents. Cleaning up the home and removing the carpet not only improved Johnny's attacks, it allowed him to grow up without relying on steroids.

The Benefits of Inhaled Steroids

A significant turning point is when a patient switches from oral steroids to inhaled steroids. This is extremely helpful, because inhaled steroids are effective at far lower doses than oral steroids. To ensure that this bridge is effective, I may have to prescribe, for a short time, up to three times the usual dose of inhaled steroids. This is still only about 3 milligrams a day in most cases. Then I will begin to reduce the amount of inhaled steroids over a period of weeks or months.

Inhaled steroids were a lifesaver for Nora, a patient of mine who was fifty-four years old and had been on 10 milligrams of oral prednisone daily for fifteen months. She had been absolutely unable to wean herself from the drug. I started her on the CAP program and reduced her dose by 1 milligram a day until she was down to 5 milligrams. We then had to slow the process a bit, reducing her by .5 milligram a day thereafter while prescribing her inhaled steroids.

Keep in mind that over the course of this time period, the patient is involved in a whole treatment program and making lifestyle changes that allow him or her to reduce medication.

Jimmy, a thirty-three-year-old banker, was on 24 puffs a day of Beclovent, an inhaled steroid, when he came to see me. He was also eating a lot of sweets and had undiagnosed hypoglycemia and sinus problems that were contributing to his ill health. We changed his diet to one emphasizing healthy proteins like fish and lean meat, complex carbohydrates like brown rice and whole wheat pastas, and healthy oils such as olive oil and flaxseed oil, rather than the hydrogenated fats and saturated fats in the foods he had been eating. This stabilized his blood sugar. His CAP program also included herbal treatments for a sinus condition, including antiinflammatory herbs like nettles, supplements such as evening primrose oil and vitamin A, and a nasal wash that I find to be very effective in sinus conditions.

A NATURAL NASAL WASH
FOR CHRONIC RHINITIS

Take a mixture of 1 teaspoon pure aloe vera gel and 1/2 teaspoon sea salt in 4 ounces of water. Aloe vera gel is a documented antiinflammatory and antibacterial agent. Salt is antibacterial and is known to reduce swelling. It can be gently inhaled into your nostrils—first tilt your head back to let the fluid fill your nasal passages and reach the back of your throat, and then blow it out. Do this twice daily.

Timing and Steroids

Here's a point that not enough physicians take seriously: the time of day when you take oral steroids can significantly reduce side effects. Steroids are produced by the body in great amounts just after waking. They drop to the lowest levels between about 2:00 and 4:00 A.M. in most people. You need to make sure the timing of the dose dovetails with your body's natural production of steroids. Take the medication when you wake up in the morning. In that way, you will mimic your body's own natural surge of steroids, and the brain will be less likely to shut down the adrenal glands. (But for patients with nighttime asthma, a nightly dose may be more effective.) Some physicians prescribe steroids in divided doses or throughout the day, but this should truly be a last resort in the most severe cases only.

How to Offset Steroid Side Effects

Any steroid-reduction program must replace the nutrients and minerals that steroids are known to deplete. I cannot emphasize the importance of this step enough. Steroids are known to cause nutritional losses, but less well-known are the impact these losses have on the body. Supplements with vitamins and minerals are absolutely crucial to any patient who has been on steroids. An overview of steroid-induced depletion follows.

Steroids deplete potassium. Hypokalemia, or loss of potassium (levels below 3.5 milligrams per deciliter of blood), can lead to congestive heart failure and heart irregularities in susceptible patients. The first sign of hypokalemia is usually muscle weakness. In severe cases, there can be total paralysis of muscles, including muscles surrounding the lungs. The highest dose of potassium available in health food stores are capsules or tablets of 99 milligrams each, and I generally recommend three a day, *though this must be carefully regulated by a physician with blood testing to monitor potassium levels.* (Too much, like too little, can be dangerous.) The use of fruits high in potassium is also helpful.

Steroids deplete protein and nitrogen. Protein depletion can lead to osteoporosis and bone fractures, as well as loss of muscle mass. When you lose protein, you also lose nitrogen, and that can lead to loss of muscle, increased pressure in the brain, and swelling in the eyes. You can improve nitrogen balance by supplementing your diet with high-quality proteins such as fish, milk, soy, and powder formulas that replenish protein.

Steroids inhibit prostaglandins, a class of potent hormone-like chemicals that control inflammation. Steroids disrupt normal pathways in the body for prostaglandins, and this can lead to peptic ulcers, impaired wound healing, kidney damage, and hormonal imbalances. Hormonal imbalances may be linked to symptoms ranging from menstrual irregularities to adrenal insufficiency to impaired growth. When steroids disrupt prostaglandins, there is no direct way to offset the damage. However, fish oils contain omega-3 fatty acids, which are known to help enhance the effects of a class of powerful, antiinflammatory prostaglandins and to block a class of prostaglandins that can cause inflammation. (See chapter 7.)

Steroids deplete calcium and magnesium. These two minerals work as a team. As one mineral flows into the cell, the other mineral flows out. The electrical balance of the cell depends on these minerals. So does muscle contraction. Supplementation with calcium citrate and magnesium citrate or magnesium aspartate can help. These forms are easily digested and assimilated. Over-supplementation with magnesium can cause diarrhea, so caution is warranted. (See chapter 7.)

Christine, a fifty-five-year-old patient of mine, had gone through menopause and was experiencing lowered bone density. She was two standard deviations below the norm on her bone density test, indicating she was at high risk for complications from osteoporosis. She was in the bottom 20 percent of the population. We weaned her off cortisone and added vitamin D, calcium, herbal treatments to gently stimulate hormone production, and an exercise program. I am pleased to say that her condition has stabilized.

Steroids have many nonspecific, damaging effects on the body. To minimize the harmful effects, it's wise to use an overall antioxidant formula. Antioxidants help the body repair cell damage and heal itself more quickly. Available at many drugstores and most health food stores, they contain vitamins A and C and beta-carotene, along with special minerals and amino acids that are known to be potent antioxidants.

SOME POINTERS ON TAPERING OFF STEROIDS

Any alteration in your prescribed medication must be supervised by a knowledgeable physician who is familiar with your history. Even so, there are some general guidelines that apply to most patients.

I've found that patients on steroids fall into three general categories: those who have been on the drug for a short term (less than a month), an intermediate term (three months to a year), or long term (up to a year or longer). These divisions are somewhat arbitrary, since each patient has an individual biochemical makeup and will respond differently to steroids, but as a rule, it is the long-term patients who suffer the most serious dependency and damaged health and who have the hardest time weaning themselves from the drug. Our goal, therefore, is to reduce medication in the safest manner possible.

Tapering off patients' prednisone use follows these general guidelines: those on high doses (above 30 milligrams a day) move to low doses (below 10 milligrams a day); those on split (twice daily) doses, to daily doses; and those on daily doses, to alternate-day doses. Depending on the patient, this is done over a period of weeks or months. I assess three factors in determining how slowly to wean a patient off steroids:

1. severity of symptoms, particularly their inability to sleep
2. severity of the patients' asthma
3. the amount of time the patient has been on steroids.

If a patient comes to me on very high amounts of steroids (over 30 milligrams a day), I will try to cut that amount by half almost immediately. Surprising as it sounds, most patients can tolerate dropping from high to moderate doses. It's when they try to go to low doses or eliminate steroids completely that they most often begin to suffer.

Take a recent patient of mine, John, a forty-five-year-old telephone executive, who came to me on 60 milligrams of prednisone a day. I cut his dose to 30 milligrams within a week by dropping the dose by 5 milligrams a day. Below 30 milligrams, the course was slower. We reduced his dose by 5 milligrams every four days until 15 milligrams a day was reached. At that point, we switched to alternate-day doses without reducing total steroids—thus prescribing 30 milligrams every other day.

This was an important moment. Even though John was receiving the same amount of the drug (30 milligrams every other day compared to 15 milligrams a day), skipping a day sends a crucial signal to the body. It tells the body the input of steroids is not constant, and so the body begins to make its own. It also allows the body a free day to recover from the side effects of the drug.

I then continued reducing the alternate-day dose by 5 milligrams every four days, until John was down to 15 milligrams every other day. At this point, it is important not to reduce drug levels too rapidly. Once we reach 5 milligrams every other day, the patient can then go off the drug.

In some rare cases, where a patient has been on high doses of steroids for years, the reduction plan may go as slowly as 5 milligrams every month. I've seen this happen once or twice. Usually the process is quicker. If, while reducing steroids, you feel unusually fatigued or suffer from rapid heartbeat and mental confusion, let your doctor know. These may be signs that you are tapering off the drug too quickly.

One possible treatment that may in the future help wean patients off cortisone is a hormone called DHEA (dehydroepiandrosterone). In postmenopausal asthma patients DHEA levels have been found to be too low, according to a 1996 study in the *Journal of Allergy and Clinical Immunology*. It is a weak steroid itself, produced in the adrenal gland. It is also a precursor hormone—a building block for other hormones, such as estrogen and testosterone. It has shown cortisone-sparing effects in lupus, and other possible uses are being investigated.

THEOPHYLLINE

A patient whose asthma was, in her own words, "totally out of control" consulted me recently. She was having attacks every day. She was also suffering from nausea, vomiting, and an inability to concentrate. Questioning revealed that she was taking theophylline. When I tested her blood levels of theophylline, they were perilously elevated.

Some doctors give theophylline to their patients without informing them about how dangerous the drug truly is, what the side effects are, when they should take it, and the serious interactions that can occur with certain drugs, or even with coffee, which has a similar effect and contains similar chemicals. One patient of mine, a twenty-one-year-old, had normal blood levels of theophylline when she first came to see me, but was suffering from signs of toxicity. She was jittery and disoriented. I found that she was drinking five or six cups of coffee a day, pushing her over the edge.

What Is Theophylline?

Theophylline belongs to a class of chemicals called methylated xanthines. These chemicals are found in coffee, tea, and chocolate. They stimulate the central nervous system and the heart—a property that can be a significant problem for patients. They also relax smooth muscles, especially those muscles that go into spasm during an asthma attack. Theophylline also works as a diuretic and helps suppress the edema (swelling) that often occurs in inflamed lung tissue.

The mechanism of theophylline has been debated for years. Scientists are still not quite sure how theophylline works. It may change the way calcium enters and leaves muscle cells (remember, calcium helps cells contract), and may inhibit a class of prostaglandins that cause inflammation. It's likely that theophylline works through several pathways in the body.

Side Effects of Theophylline

Theophylline is a powerful and, in my opinion, often toxic medication. However, studies do show that low doses, below the so-called therapeutic range, may be helpful, while "therapeutic" levels can be dangerous. Side effects include nervousness, the jitters, nausea, vomiting, tachycardia (racing heart), and palpitations. Toxic levels can cause insomnia, vomiting, diarrhea, convulsions, and coma. Theophylline, even in low doses, is particularly dangerous to patients who suffer from serious liver problems. That's because theophylline passes through the liver, and if it is not metabolized and broken down, it stays at high levels in the blood and is not excreted. The drug can easily reach toxic levels. However, when properly monitored, this medication can help a patient through a difficult period.

Studies have linked theophylline to learning disorders and disabilities, and many patients report that the drug makes them feel extremely agitated. I examined one child on theophylline who was suffering from hyperactivity and learning disorders. He was taking 100 milligrams of Theo-Dur (a brand of theophylline) two times a day and was continually sick. When we cleaned up his environment and gave him an air purifier, a whole range of antiinflammatory and antioxidant supplements, and sprays using an at-home spacer (see the instructions for using sprays, page 116), he began to do very well. After three months he was off the Theo-Dur and back in school on a regular basis. His hyperactivity vanished.

A note for the elderly: as you age, it becomes harder to detoxify and metabolize drugs efficiently. One sixty-five-year-old man came to me. He had suffered from asthma for many years and had been prescribed theophylline. However, the theophylline made him jittery, so he was also given Valium. The Valium made him sleepy, so he drank coffee. As he aged, his body was less efficient at metabolizing these medications, and by the time he came to me, he was toxic—overtired and tense at the same time. Reducing his medications produced a sharp improvement.

Substances That Interfere with Theophylline

Smoke. People who smoke metabolize theophylline at twice the rate of the average person, so their dose needs to be higher than normal.

Protein. Individuals who eat a high-protein, low-carbohydrate diet metabolize theophylline at a 25 percent faster rate than normal.

Carbohydrate. A low-protein, high-carbohydrate diet has the opposite effect: it slows down metabolism by 25 percent.

Infection. During viral infections or fevers, theophylline is metabolized more slowly than usual.

Vaccines. Flu vaccines increase the absorption of theophylline.

Caffeine. Coffee increases the levels of theophylline in the blood.

Inderal. This heart disease drug slows theophylline metabolism, so the dose must be lowered.

Other drugs. Tagamet, a common ulcer medication, increases the absorption of theophylline. Nicotine, including a nicotine patch, may increase theophylline levels. So do certain antibiotics, like erythromycin and a newer class of antibiotics called quinolones (both are commonly prescribed for asthmatics when they suffer from respiratory infections).

In addition, theophylline itself affects two other drugs. Lithium (taken for manic-depression) is eliminated quickly from the body when a patient takes theophylline. Phenytoin, an anticonvulsant, does not work as well in the presence of theophylline.

How and When Should You Take Theophylline?

There is one problem with doses of theophylline: it is an extremely difficult drug to administer properly because it has to stay within an extremely narrow dosage range to be both effective and safe. The difference between an effective and a toxic dose is terrifyingly small. Even when doses are too low to be effective, side effects may still occur.

Another difficulty with theophylline is that many substances can interfere with its absorption, and so actual blood levels are unpredictable on a day-to-day basis. For instance, food enhances the absorption of theophylline, so asthmatics who skip breakfast may not be getting the full benefit of the drug. One patient of mine had been doing just that for years: skipping breakfast. At night, however, she took her evening dose with a big meal, and the drug was absorbed into her system immediately. She had no idea why, every night, she felt jittery and sick from the drug. The fact is, her dinner dose was too high.

If your physician does prescribe theophylline, he or she must first establish the correct dosage. Doctors are taught to take two blood tests every four days until there is no variation in blood levels. Many doctors, obviously, do not monitor the drug this closely because of the practical difficulty. Yet all patients on theophylline should have periodic blood tests to monitor blood levels of the drug.

Prescribing the drug is just as complex. Your physician must decide what type to give you: short-acting (peaking within two hours of ingestion), intermediate (peaking in four hours), or long-acting (lasting sixteen hours and staying in the body for two or three days). The rate of absorption differs between sustained-release and shorter-acting theophylline, and among different brands. Generic versions of the drug are not recommended, since they may vary in potency by as much as 25 percent. That means there is no standard dose for any particular form or brand of the drug.

I do not recommend theophylline very often. Any drug with such potential toxicity and such stringent requirements for continually measuring blood levels leaves me wary and concerned. The older forms of theophylline—the drugs Marax and Tedral—have fallen out of favor today, because they could not be individually monitored.

I prefer a version of theophylline like Slo-phyllin, because the dosage is accurately delivered in a time-released fashion so that patients don't get sharp bursts of medication.

COMMON FORMS OF THEOPHYLLINE

Aminophylline. Sold as Aminophylline tablets or Aminophylline oral liquid.

Oxtriphylline. Sold as Choledyl SA tablets. The tablets are sustained release.

Theophylline—short acting. Sold as Marax tablets and Quibron tablets.

Theophylline—sustained release. Sold as Slo-Phyllin tablets, Aerolate capsules, Theolair tablets, Slo-bid Gyrocaps, Quibron-T/SR tablets, Slo-Phyllin Gyrocaps, Theo-Dur tablets, Theo-24, Uni-Dur tablets, and Uniphyl tablets.

Theophylline—liquids. Sold as Aerolate liquid, Elixophyllin elixir, Slo-Phyllin 80 syrup, Theoclear-80 syrup, Theolair liquid.

Some Tips on Reducing Theophylline

How does theophylline work?

We don't know. However, at low doses it seems to exhibit antiinflammatory ability. At higher doses, it eases movement in the diaphragm. It seems to enhance lung capacity and increase oxygen levels in the lung. Therefore, the key to reducing this drug is achieving those effects naturally. That's why breathing exercises are extremely important, along with proper nutrition. In the context of a program like CAP, every aspect of change and treatment is dedicated to enhancing oxygen levels.

Patients on theophylline are often taking 300 milligrams twice a day. They can usually be reduced to 200 milligrams twice a day.

After two weeks, their physician should check their peak-flow-meter numbers (see chapter 13) to be sure that the patient's lung capacity is still normal. Then the drug can be further reduced to 300 milligrams at bedtime alone for two weeks, then 200 milligrams at bedtime alone for two weeks. Many patients can then go off the drug. This must be done under the supervision of a skilled physician.

Some physicians may point out that below 300 milligrams twice a day, you are not achieving therapeutic levels of the drug. I understand this. Nonetheless, with any powerful drug, you want to wean the body from the medication in a gradual, nonstressful fashion. Besides, some patients still feel better at that level of medication.

At the same time, it's a good idea to try to mimic the effects of theophylline. I teach breathing exercises to all my patients but do so immediately for patients on theophylline. It's extremely important to assist the diaphragm in moving freely. It can also be helpful to pay attention to foods and substances containing natural theophylline-like chemicals. These include caffeine, chocolate, and tea. Sometimes patients find a few cups of tea very beneficial in tiding them over the reduction period. However, caution is recommended.

Theophylline is known to disrupt and dysregulate cellular membranes and act as a diuretic, leaching fluids from the cells. Therefore, a reduction program should replenish electrolytes, which are nutrients that theophylline can deplete. This can be done by supplementing with calcium, magnesium, and potassium (for dosage levels, see chapter 7).

BETA-AGONISTS (BRONCHODILATORS)

Beta-agonist sprays, which patients usually call bronchodilators or inhalers, deserve a section all their own, because they have been the story of the last decade in asthma. They are hugely popular, extremely convenient, instantly effective, used all over the world, and now many physicians fear that it is our heavy reliance on these drugs that has caused asthma fatalities to soar. Most people don't notice any pronounced side effects—until one day the drug just doesn't work, and they simply can't breathe and are rushed to the hospital. Beta-agonists, when used improperly, may indeed be deadly.

In Europe between 1961 and 1966, for instance, when beta-agonists first became available and popular, there was a huge jump in the mortality rate of asthma. The most vulnerable group were children age ten to fourteen; according to a study in the premier British medical journal, *The Lancet,* the death rate for these youngsters increased sevenfold. One only needs to contemplate the statistics to imagine the unnecessary tragedy striking many families.

Another study conducted in the 1980s and reported in the *New England Journal of Medicine* found that not only did beta-agonist sprays increase the risk of death, certain sprays were deadlier than others. For instance, fenoterol, a long-acting beta-agonist not used in the U.S, was over twice as dangerous as albuterol. Another study in this journal found that when patients were given fenoterol regularly rather than on an as-needed basis, their asthma worsened. Yet another study found that many patients who died suddenly of asthma were taking both theophylline and beta-agonists.

Even more alarming, in January 1994 there was a recall of a generic form of the most popular beta-agonist spray, albuterol, because it was contaminated with bacteria.

Yet I do recommend they be handy for most asthmatics, to be used on an as-needed basis. Patients love beta-agonist sprays because they can banish the agony of an asthma attack in just a few moments. Not only are they convenient, they provide instant relief in a way that no other medication can.

Because patients love them so much, there's no doubt these medicines are here to stay. There are patients who absolutely refuse to leave home without their sprays. I've had more than one patient come into my office in bad shape, sneak into the bathroom and take a few puffs of a spray, and then walk up to me saying, "My asthma's bothering me a little, but it's not that bad today." Other patients tell me about their persistent fear of leaving home without their sprays. They are simply afraid to be anywhere without having their sprays handy.

I am not sanguine about the overuse of these sprays, but I do understand why patients like them. What I try to do is explain how these sprays work, why they are so appealing, and how to best avoid their dangers.

What Are Beta-Agonists?

Beta-agonists are drugs that block a receptor in airway muscle cells called the beta-receptor. There are two types of beta-receptors, beta-1 and beta-2. Beta-1 is common in the heart, and drugs that help relax the heart muscle are known as beta-blockers. Beta-2 is common in airway muscles. Beta-agonist sprays primarily affect beta-2 receptors, dilating and opening the lungs, but they also affect beta-1 receptors in the heart. That's why these sprays inevitably speed up the heart and, at the same time, cause blood pressure to drop slightly. They may also cause restlessness and muscle tremors, headaches, and anxiety.

Beta-blockers can sometimes be contraindicated, so caution should be used in taking them. One sixty-eight-year-old heart patient of mine had trouble when he took beta-agonist sprays. For his heart problem, I switched him to a calcium channel blocker. For his asthma, I prescribed other medications, and his heart symptoms improved.

There are seven major types of beta-agonists: isoetharine, metaproterenol, terbutaline, perbuterol, albuterol, and bitolterol. The seventh, fenoterol, was never available here and has fallen out of favor because of the deaths associated with its use, particularly in New Zealand, where it was a popular drug. A new beta-agonist, salmeterol, has just been approved in this country.

Common Side Effects of Beta-Agonists

Patients often notice that sprays are marvelously effective for the first few weeks and then lose some of their potency. That's because after a few weeks of taking beta-agonists, the airway receptors become less sensitive to the drug. It may also be due to the fact that if patients don't shake the canister properly, they will be getting a lot of medication when it is full, and less as they begin to use it up. Also, some patients do not spray into the back of the throat, and particles may settle on the tongue and be swallowed, leading to systemic effects. One patient of mine found that if she simply rinsed her mouth out after spraying, side effects were lessened.

Clearly, the most significant danger of beta-agonists is overuse of the drugs. A Canadian study showed that excess use (twenty-five or more of the small canisters a year) of salbutamol, a drug recently approved in the United States, increased risk of death forty times.

Lewis Kohl, deputy director of the Department of Emergency Medicine at Kings County Hospital in New York, zeroes in on the danger of beta-agonists: "One of the critical factors when someone starts to get tight and really sick," he told me in an interview, "is that by taking bronchodilators, they are causing the blood flow to increase and blood vessels to dilate. Beta-agonists also dilate blood vessels as well as the airways themselves, but in severe cases the airways take longer to open. So what you've got is increased blood flow without increased oxygen. It's called a ventilation-perfusion mismatch, and what it means on the bottom line is that you get starved for oxygen. Those with heart disease and asthma are placed in particular danger. Follow this rule:

if you are pounding on your puffer, you need an emergency room or your doctor."

Instead of making the patient better in a dangerous situation, these drugs can be depriving him of oxygen. Blood is flowing in the vessels in the lungs, but it's not absorbing enough oxygen. Remember, the lungs are very dynamic. People think of them like two big balloons, but they are really a series of about 2 million little balloons. And those 2 million balloons are losing oxygen.

"Doctors have written about this problem," notes Kohl, "but it's often not recognized clinically. People who are smart about asthma know it happens. You're spraying someone with a heart stimulant that may actually be taking oxygen away from the heart. It's a jolt to the body. Now, this is not a problem for the average person taking a routine amount of spray, but when someone gets into trouble, bronchodilator therapy alone can be truly dangerous."

No wonder, then, that when a patient begins to overdose on the spray, the result can be a terrifying rebound reaction. Called "locked lung syndrome," it is a state of bronchospasm that may be hard to break. One result can be death.

For someone in serious distress, Kohl's solution is completely different—a nebulizer propelled by oxygen so that the patient is getting a high concentration of oxygen along with the medicine. (Nebulizers are machines that turn liquid medication into a fine mist that is easily breathed in.) Corticosteroids may be unavoidable in these situations. The key is not to get to this point.

All beta-agonists cause some shakiness, because the beta-receptors in muscles are affected along with those in the lung. Some drugs are targeted primarily for the lungs and cause fewer side effects. In general, beta-agonists can cause changes in heart rate and are not recommended for patients with heart problems of any kind. One seventy-four-year-old patient of mine was so sensitive that his heart rate jumped to 150 beats a minute after 2 puffs of Ventolin.

Beta-agonists should also be used with caution in patients who suffer from hyperthyroidism or diabetes. Overuse of these drugs has been associated with fatal asthma attacks, perhaps due to a drug-induced heart attack caused by hypokalemia, or lowered blood potassium. Overuse can also lead to what is known as "paradoxical bronchospasm," or in essence, a severe asthma attack. Patients may also experience muscle tremors, nervousness, palpitations, chest pain, racing heart, insomnia, irritable behavior, vomiting, and stomachache.

Here are some common sprays that are available, their brand names, and their effects:

Albuterol is probably the most popular spray in this country. Although a 1995 study found that albuterol worsened attention deficit disorder (ADD) in children, it causes less shakiness than the other sprays. Albuterol goes by the brand name of Proventil or Ventolin. Typical dosage is 2 puffs four times a day. The spray's effects are immediate and last from four to six hours.

Terbutaline is known as Brethine, Brethaire, or Bricanyl and is a popular spray that, like albuterol, is instantly effective. It lasts four to six hours. Patients have a tendency to develop drug tolerance with terbutaline, so that effects are less marked as time goes on. Like albuterol, it can cause shakiness. Terbutaline is the only beta-agonist approved for use during pregnancy.

Isoproterenol, known as Isuprel, is not as popular as it once was, because it is not as specific a beta-2 blocker as newer medications. It stimulates the heart and intensifies the contractions, so it can be dangerous for asthmatics with heart problems. Nonetheless, it is sometimes used in emergency rooms in severe attacks and has even been used intravenously in some cases.

Isoetharine, known as Bronkosol or Bronkometer, is immediately effective and lasts only about an hour. It has a tendency to cause rapid heartbeat and muscle tremors. It is one of the less popular sprays, but it is still used fairly frequently for children.

Perbuterol, known as Maxair, is a fairly common beta-agonist with side effects like the others, but it is a bit longer lasting. Doses are usually every four to six hours.

Metaproterenol, known as Alupent or Metaprel, works instantly and lasts for two to four hours (shorter than some of the other sprays). It stimulates the heart less than terbutaline or albuterol, but it also does not act as directly on the lungs. This drug interacts with certain antidepressants (known as tricyclic and MAO inhibitors).

Fenoterol is a long-acting medication that was popular in New Zealand and parts of Europe but fell out of favor before it could become available here because of the high mortality rate associated with it. It is believed to severely deplete potassium, leading to cardiac arrest. Thank goodness we missed this one.

Salmeterol, recently approved in this country, is a quick-acting and long-lasting beta-agonist spray. It has shown good results so far in patients with well-controlled asthma, allowing patients to manage their asthma through the night. It is, however, inefficient for acute asthma attacks and in some cases has contributed to deaths. A letter to the *New England Journal of Medicine* reported that two elderly patients were found dead, holding their inhalers. Patients who are not properly instructed in the use of these drugs may mistakenly use them for short-term relief of acute attacks. Because they are long-lasting drugs and take at least half an hour to provide relief, improper use could result in a fatal asthma attack.

When to Use Beta-Agonist Sprays

The safest approach is to use sprays on an intermittent, as-needed basis, when an acute attack threatens. Careful rinsing of your mouth after each usage can reduce side effects. Regular use of sprays provides symptomatic relief while allowing a serious underlying disease to continue unabated.

Some Tips for Reducing Beta-Agonist Usage

Weaning patients from regular use of beta-agonist sprays is much easier than steroids or theophylline, though once again it needs to be done in the context of a complete program and under physician supervision. For instance, if an asthmatic patient is taking 4 puffs twice a day, I will reduce them to 2 puffs three times a day, then down to 2 puffs in the morning and evening, and then on an as-needed basis. This can usually be accomplished in the first six weeks.

Tapering doses of beta-agonists is done much the same way as weaning a patient from steroids or theophylline: the CAP program is begun, and when the patient is stabilized, the dose is reduced.

One important point about beta-agonists: often patients are "addicted" to the feeling they get from the sprays, and to the sense of safety they feel. In actuality, if a patient tests their peak-flow-meter levels, they may find that many times when they feel as if they need a spray, they are actually in the safe range of lung function and can go without.

HOW TO SPRAY

Believe it or not, half the asthma patients I see do not know how to properly administer their inhalers and sprays, and a recent study found that only 4 percent of women use these sprays correctly, as compared to 43 percent of men. In addition, patients often forget to note the time of their last dose. I've seen patients spray their medication on their tongues and swallow it, resulting, in some cases, in systemic effects like shakiness and nausea. Other patients spray the medication and instantly breathe it out through their mouths and noses. Still others breathe out when they should breathe in, leaving a cloud of medication in the air, or they don't shake their inhalers vigorously before each use, so that they end up with variable amounts of medication, rather than a properly metered dose.

Follow the steps below to properly medicate yourself with a spray, being sure to first shake the canister well:

1. Open your mouth.
2. Exhale.
3. Place the canister an inch from your mouth.
4. Spray toward the back of your throat.
5. As you spray, inhale deeply.
6. Hold the breath for up to ten seconds so that the spray can disperse evenly throughout the lungs. Take your time, then exhale.
7. If your doctor instructs you to take 2 puffs, wait up to 5 minutes between puffs. Each puff is an individual dose of medication.
8. After spraying, clean your container, so that dust and particles don't seep into it. Keep the cover on when the spray is not in use, so that you don't inhale dust particles. (One child inhaled a paper clip that had found its way into the spray canister.)
9. In cases where the patient has acute asthma, take one dose of the spray, wait fifteen minutes, and then take another dose. This gives the lungs the opportunity to open in response to the first dose, and can be more effective.

I recommend that my patients use spacers when they can. A spacer (available at any pharmacy by prescription) is a small tube attached to the mouthpiece of the spray canister. This tube increases the distance from spray to mouth and allows the particles of medication to separate, so that smaller molecules reach the lungs. These smaller molecules penetrate lung tissue more deeply. Spacers also allow more spray to be inhaled directly, rather than falling in droplets on the tongue, so they tend to decrease fungal infections when steroid sprays are used. A spacer is especially helpful for children, because they may not inhale at the right time, and it gives them a chance to inhale a few times while the medication travels through the spacer tube. Spacers range from simple tubes to accordion-like devices.

Just as effective for home use is a nebulizer, which is one of the most underutilized and important devices available for asthma. Turning liquid medication into a fine mist, nebulizers allow asthmatics to control their aerosol therapy. One benefit of nebulizers is that they allow you to use pure medication without any of the extra chemicals often included in aerosol sprays. Nebulizers are quite helpful for children, as well as some adults, because they allow you to slowly absorb medication at a controlled pace.

ADRENALINE AND ADRENALINE-LIKE DRUGS

Like beta-agonist bronchodilators, adrenaline (also known as epinephrine) and ephedrine are drugs that belong to a class of substances that stimulate the beta-receptors in the nervous system, lungs, and heart. Their problem is that they are nonspecific. They not only affect the lungs but strongly constrict muscles surrounding arteries and smooth veins, as well as muscles around the bladder. Adrenaline can cause a sense of panic because it stimulates the nervous system so strongly. The side effects can be unpleasant and sometimes dangerous. Nonetheless, adrenaline is almost always used when an asthmatic reaches the hospital.

If you are given a shot of adrenaline, expect to feel shaky

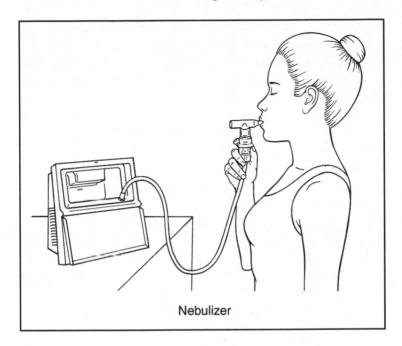

Nebulizer

as your breathing improves. You will feel relief within minutes. However, because adrenaline is quickly destroyed in the body, its effect may not be sufficient to relieve symptoms. You may need another shot in twenty minutes. The usual dose of adrenaline is .2 to .3 milliliters injected under the skin, with a maximum of three doses.

Adrenaline, as you may know, is produced naturally in your body by the adrenal glands in response to stress. Injecting adrenaline gives the body an artificial and instant burst. Adrenaline guns up the nervous system and opens the airways.

Another useful form of adrenaline is known as EpiPen. I recommend that any patient suffering from severe asthma keep this with them at all times. It's an injectable form of adrenaline in a container that looks like a small pen. You can administer it yourself in an emergency—and of course, I recommend it in emergencies only, but it can save lives. If you suffer a sudden and severe asthma attack, you can self-administer epinephrine on the way to the hospital. You press the tip of the pen against your thigh or arm, and it injects a dose rather painlessly.

Because adrenaline is generally used in emergencies, it is not a drug that most patients become dependent on, and so I do not need to provide them with a reducing schedule. However, I do see asthma patients who are hospitalized regularly and come to rely on adrenaline shots as a method of treatment. If you have been hospitalized even once and needed adrenaline, you are a prime candidate for a comprehensive treatment program like the one outlined in this book.

ANTIHISTAMINES

These are a common class of drugs that are often prescribed for asthma and that I dispense when my own patients are suffering an acute exacerbation of asthma induced by allergies (by seasonal pollens, for instance, or exposure to cats or dogs). The four most common ones prescribed today are Seldane, Claritin, Hismanil, and Zertic. Because none of these drugs cross the blood-brain barrier, they do not enter the brain and therefore do not cause the kind of fatigue and tiredness commonly associated with older antihistamines like chlortrimeton. Unlike other antihistamines, Claritin does not interact with the drugs erythromycin or ketoconazole.

Caution should be used in taking antihistamines daily over the long term. Recent animal research found that antihistamines like Hismanil potentiated cancer growth. Although this finding may not be applicable to humans, it is wise to be careful until we know more. In addition, antihistamines may not be helpful to those asthmatics who are already fatigued or depressed, since many of these medications intensify fatigue.

CROMOLYN SODIUM AND NEDOCROMIL SODIUM

Cromolyn sodium is a nontoxic medication with strong antiinflammatory properties and virtually no significant side effects. It has been available in this country since 1975, and its popularity is steadily growing.

Cromolyn sodium, known as Intal, is invaluable in asthma (as well as in allergic rhinitis, or sinus conditions) because it stabilizes the mast cell. The mast cell is one of the primary cells involved in the allergic cascade: when a mast cell is stimulated, it bursts, releasing histamine and triggering other inflammatory substances. Cromolyn sodium not only stabilizes the mast cells, it seems to reduce the sensitivity of the airways in general.

The beauty of this drug is that it inhibits both early- and late-phase asthma reactions (as explained in chapter 5). This means that cromolyn sodium can, when given over time, prevent the acute asthmatic reaction. But it also, over time, will help relieve the delayed inflammation known as the late-phase. This medication not only helps allergic asthma, it can relieve exercise-induced asthma, as well as asthma caused by cold or foggy weather. It's a truly exciting medication because it works so well with so few side effects.

Are there any drawbacks to this drug? A few. First, though it can prevent an acute attack if it is used before a person is exposed to an allergen, it does not relieve acute attacks once they have begun. In fact, it may worsen the condition in some sensitive individuals by causing local irritation. Bronchodilators are effective in such cases.

Intal also has minor side effects. Occasionally patients complain about throat irritation, cough, or dry mouth after using the medication. This may be due to its powdery nature. It is also to be used with caution in patients with liver or kidney disease, because the drug is metabolized in those two organs.

Compare those side effects to the panoply of side effects and fatalities associated with other popular drugs, and there is no question that cromolyn sodium should be used more frequently for asthma, though not during the onset of an acute attack.

Cromolyn sodium used to be manufactured as a dry powder in capsule form and had to be used with a special inhaler. Now it is available as a convenient spray.

The major problem patients have with cromolyn sodium is that it does not always work as quickly and dramatically as other medications. Though some patients may find instant relief with the drug, others may not notice relief for up to six weeks. For asthma patients who are wheezing daily, that can seem too long a time. They become discouraged and need to be reminded that with a little patience they may find that this drug works beautifully.

The medication is particularly loved by patients who suffer from intermittent allergic asthma. When such a patient knows they will be exposed to an allergen—dog dander at a relative's, for instance—they can treat themselves with the drug before contact with marvelous results. Patients can also begin treating themselves a week before hay fever season.

The usual dosage of Intal is 2 puffs, four times a day, for a total of 80 milligrams a day. If a patient is having trouble inhaling the medication, I will sometimes recommend using a bronchodilating spray first, so that the airways are open and can fully absorb the cromolyn sodium.

Another related drug that has just been released in the United States is nedocromil sodium, called Tilade. Tilade seems to inhibit inflammatory chemicals, not just in mast cells, but in a whole range of cells, including eosinophils, macrophages, platelets, and neutrophils. Potent inflammatory chemicals, such as histamines, prostaglandins, and leukotrienes, are blocked. Tilade is not absorbed systemically, and initial studies indicate that it may be as effective as Intal. Thus far, the drug seems to have minimal side effects.

ZILEUTON AND INTERLEUKIN INHIBITORS

A whole new class of drugs is currently being studied and is now available. They interrupt the inflammatory cascade very early in the process, at the cellular level, and in very specific ways. Zileuton, is one such drug, due to become available in 1997. Preliminary clinical studies show the drug to be extremely effective; however, a troubling rise in liver enzymes has put this medication on hold. Another drug, Accolate, has been deemed safe by the F.D.A. but prior to approval it had been sent back after it was found to cause an increase in the blood levels of other common medications. At this point just be careful since Aspirin and Cumidin can potentiate this drug. Many other drugs can be antagonistic to this drug including Erythromycin and Theophylline. According to a recent article in the *Wall Street Journal*, the effort to produce the first new asthma medication in twenty-five years "has been marked by failure, delays, and the unsettling worry that the new drugs pose unacceptable risks for long-term users, especially children."

Expect these drugs to come to market in the years to come. They are interleukin inhibitors. Interleukins can cause inflammation and are released very early in the inflammatory process. Scientists are hoping to get closer and closer to the actual first point of inflammation, even to the information about inflammation that is processed in the gene itself.

I am very interested in this line of research, but I also feel great caution. Many new "miracle" drugs turn out, when used by the public at large, to have serious side effects. James Fish, M.D., of the Thomas Jefferson Medical College in Philadelphia has said, "None of these drugs cures asthma." The new drugs will come in pill form.

Nobody likes to be sick. Any human being with a chronic illness wants relief from the burden of daily discomfort. So it's understandable that we turn to prescription drugs in an attempt to regain a sense of well-being. But as I have tried to make alarmingly clear in this chapter, medications often mask the underlying problem in asthma without treating it. You can feel better without relying solely on drugs. With your physician's careful supervision, you can soon reach a point where you use drugs minimally and cease to regard them as the core of your asthma treatment.

Although my guidelines have been included in this chapter, I want to emphasize one last time that this is one part of my program you cannot conduct on your own. No patient should change their dosage or medication without the supervision of a skilled physician.

I also want you to understand that weaning yourself from reliance on medications is a step that works only in the context of a complete and sweeping program like CAP. If you decide to try this program, you, like most of my patients, will be astonished that you are so comfortably able to reduce or eliminate medications that you have been taking for years.

DOCTOR'S RECOMMENDATIONS FOR ACTION

1. In consultation with your doctor, determine which medications, if any, are appropriate for you. When used properly, medications are an invaluable tool. However, many

asthma patients are overmedicated. Prescriptions for asthma medications have tripled since 1972, and these powerful medications can cause side effects that impair health. I recommend that most of my patients taper off drugs—and you can, too, but it must be done under a doctor's strict supervision.

2. Any drug-tapering program needs to be carried out in the context of a program like CAP, in which lifestyle and environment are being changed and the body is being nourished with highly nutritious, nonallergenic foods and specific nutrients. Only in this way can you repair years of damage due to chronic illness and overmedication.

3. Steroids can be lifesavers in acute and potentially fatal attacks, but if a patient needs steroids, that is a wake-up call. Don't take steroid use lightly.

4. Patients must be weaned from steroids carefully by their physician. They can be switched from oral to inhaled steroids and then gently tapered off inhaled steroids.

5. All drugs have side effects, but patients are often not informed about those side effects. Be aware of the side effects of the drugs you are taking. Let your doctor know if you are experiencing any of the side effects so dosages can be readjusted.

6. Be careful when using beta-agonists. They expand the bronchial tubes during acute attacks but do not treat the underlying inflammation. Therefore, they can give symptom control while asthma silently worsens. For this reason, overuse of beta-agonists can cause susceptibility to fatal asthma attacks.

7. Know the best time of day to take your drugs for maximum effect. Be aware of foods and drugs that interfere with the action of your medications—either limiting or enhancing their effect. Learn exactly how to use your inhaler for maximum effectiveness.

8. Choose antiinflammatory medications like Intal or

Tilade rather than cortisone if possible. They have very few side effects and are tolerated well by many patients.

9. Children require special care in determining correct medication. They can benefit from the use of spacers and nebulizers.

CHAPTER SEVEN

How Healing Begins: Super Nutrients

It began when I was nine years old," Kris, the young woman in my office, said. "My family was on a ski vacation in Colorado, and we kept running from ski slopes into the hot tub. Suddenly I couldn't breathe, and I had to go to the hospital. Since then, I've been hospitalized almost every year, and I feel like I'm addicted to my medications."

Kris is twenty-four years old, a model by profession, waifishly slender and elegant, but when she first came to see me, she had not been able to work in six months.

"Last January I was running around from five in the morning to seven at night doing print modeling, and then one night, I woke up and couldn't breathe, and my inhaler just didn't work," she told me. "I kept taking puffs and I still couldn't breathe. It was terrifying. I was hospitalized for five days.

"The doctor said he couldn't believe I let myself get that sick, but I hate doctors and hospitals. When they give you a shot of adrenaline, you feel horrible, like you're speeding and yet you're a million miles away. There's this roar of nurses and doctors around you, but you're so disoriented you can't understand what they're saying. And then they pump you up with antibiotics and steroids. The steroids make you feel so out of control, like hyperactive.

"I've been in and out of emergency rooms and each time they just send me home with a handful of medications. I feel completely frustrated. I have to think about my asthma all the time. I can't even laugh without coughing. I don't go to parties anymore, because people smoke and I just can't deal with not breathing for the next few days."

Kris's story is not unusual. Asthma calls into play the intricacies of the immune and nervous systems, which are profoundly linked by a vast web of chemical messengers. That's one reason asthma can be triggered by so many factors—from foods to pollutants, changes in temperature, stress, allergens, and unsuspected toxins anywhere from the bedroom to the boardroom. All these stresses strain the body, leading to nutritional deficiencies and cellular damage.

In Kris's case, nutritional supplements were crucial to regaining her health. Her diet had been poor for years. She ate on the fly—slices of pizza, hamburgers, and Diet Cokes. She took no vitamin supplements, and her tests showed that she was deficient in magnesium as well as most B vitamins.

"It worked so quickly, I was amazed," she said, referring to her nutritional supplementation. "At first I felt kind of strange because I was taking loads of vitamins, but within two weeks I felt great, I had more energy, I didn't have trouble breathing, I could even walk down the street and go up and down steps without feeling out of breath. I have to go to lots of appointments all day long, so feeling better made a world of difference. Now I'm sleeping well, not always waking up at night. My overall health has been so much better, and I'm more even-keeled emotionally, too. I used to get sick and feel sorry for myself, then get better and party, then get sick again. Now I'm off that merry-go-round."

Nutritional deficiencies are an important key to beginning to heal asthma. Nutrient supplementation targets asthma at a cellular level, where I believe things first go wrong.

How do you work at the cellular level? You study what happens to cells in the lung during an asthma attack. What inflammatory chemicals are released? What damage is caused to the body? What nutrients are required by the body to repair that damage?

During an asthma attack, an allergen or toxin causes an inflammatory response in the lungs. That response actually triggers a whole avalanche of inflammatory chemicals that attack not only the invader but also the tissue at the site of the invasion, attempting through inflammation to confine it and then kill it. As I've explained, perhaps the most damaging by-products of inflammation are free radicals, highly reactive, highly charged particles that can wreak havoc and cause cell damage.

Unless you have a rich supply of antioxidants that can quench those free radicals, you will be unable to prevent tissue damage. Over the long term, that damage can lead to a lung that is scarred, fibrotic, and perpetually inflamed.

THE NUTRACEUTICAL REVOLUTION

Nutrition is not the only answer to asthma, but it is a cornerstone, perhaps the most important one. A few supplements will not miraculously banish your asthma, but supplementation can make all the difference when applied in the context of a complete program. In fact, I don't believe asthmatics can get truly well without nutrient replenishment, either through diet or supplementation.

I have found that nutritional therapy can have a powerful impact on the course of asthma. Research backs me up. The nutrients that work in real life asthmatics have been proven in the laboratory to alter inflammation at a cellular level and help the body to repair itself. I treat asthma with supplements designed to accomplish two goals: to slow and dampen inflammation and to help the body repair itself.

There is a gathering mountain of evidence that nutrients can improve overall health. Nevertheless—and this is an extremely important point—they cannot undo the damage of an unhealthy lifestyle. A recent study of 29,000 Finnish men aged fifty to sixty-nine who were heavy smokers with a high-fat diet showed no benefit from taking the nutrients beta-carotene and vitamin E for six years. Those who quit smoking did show benefit. The study raised questions: Do healthy foods rich in nutrients provide unknown nutritional cofactors that prevent disease? Are higher amounts of nutrients, taken for a longer period of time, necessary to improve health in an individual leading a toxic lifestyle?

This particular study does not negate the fact that many epidemiological studies demonstrate a strong link between nutrients and health although they do not prove a cause-and-effect relationship. Two important epidemiological studies of nearly 120,000 people found a significant reduction in heart disease among men and women who took daily supplements of vitamin E. A study of 22,000 male doctors found protective benefit from taking 50 milligrams of beta-carotene every other day for a decade. Another study showed that 9 out of 10 doctors approve the use of antioxidants for chronic heart disease. There are over fifteen studies to date showing that individuals with a diet rich in carotene reduce their risk of lung cancer. Carotenoids have also been linked to protection against heart disease and strokes. One molecule of beta-carotene has been shown to regulate nearly 16 billion free-radical reactions.

Nutrients with antioxidant properties are an equally rich and exciting source of promising studies. Studies done at universities in Texas and California found that vitamins C and E can prevent the oxidation of "bad" LDL cholesterol. A study of 3,000 Swiss men found that the risk of death from cancer was significantly higher among men with low levels of carotene and vitamin C in their blood. Other studies have shown that women with precancerous changes of the cervix had low levels of the same two vitamins.

Given the avalanche of studies about nutrients and health, it's not surprising that a special term has been coined for this burgeoning new field of nutritional medicine. *Nutraceutical*—nutrients that may fight and prevent illness—has become a buzzword of late. Articles on healing nutrients, from vitamins to phytochemicals (plant chemicals), have appeared in the last few years on the covers of magazines like *Time* and *Newsweek* and in articles in *The New York Times*. Even a publication like *American Druggist* ran a cover story on plant remedies in May 1992.

Research on the capacity of plant substances to prevent tumors is a hot new field that makes headlines in national media and is now considered a viable topic for publication in top medical journals. This is an intriguing new field that is providing fresh insight into new treatments for illness.

The American public seems to be taking to heart the new research. In 1993 alone, sales of vitamin E supplements soared by 39 percent (to $123 million); beta-carotene sales jumped 31 percent (to $22 million); and vitamin C sales rose 10 percent (to $117 million).

As a nutritionally oriented physician, I feel that one of the most important medical advances of this century is our new understanding that nutrients can have profound benefits for our health. But perhaps the most important news we have is that nature's healing capacities are both complex and subtle. Foods contain far more than vitamins, minerals, protein, carbohydrates, and fats.

IT'S TIME TO CHANGE OUR SIMPLISTIC THINKING

The very concept of vitamins and minerals now turns out to be a simplistic one. *Vitamin* was originally coined from the Latin *vita* ("life") and the *amine* (a scientific term that means "containing amino acids"). Vitamins do not, however, contain amino acids, which are the building blocks of protein. The loose definition of a vitamin is an organic substance present in foods and essential to nutrition in man.

Minerals, in turn, are considered inorganic substances obtained by mining, and the word was coined from the Latin *minerale* ("ore"). Minerals are important as cofactors in most reactions in our bodies. Hormones, another classic concept, originally meant substances secreted into the blood and regulating organ systems and tissues.

It turns out that none of these substances can be easily classified. They are staggeringly complex.

Consider hormones. Plants are known to contain substances that act like hormones in our body, filling up the same receptor sites. In addition, some hormones can be created in the blood, kidneys, lungs, and other tissues. Some vitamins, such as vitamin E, function as regulators of hormones, and vitamin E can combat excess levels of estrogen in women. Vitamin B_6, in turn, has been shown in some cases to help potentiate progesterone in women deficient in that hormone. Vitamin D is transformed by the body into vitamin D_3, a hormone-like substance that is crucial in the formation of bone. Most vitamins and minerals play a wide variety of roles in the body, assisting virtually every action and reaction, working as cofactors in enzyme reactions, as building blocks for new tissue and bone, as antioxidants that clean up free-radical damage.

There are countless other substances that also improve health. Some are amino acids, such as carnitine, glutamine, and cysteine, to name a few. They can have profound beneficial effects on health. Sulforaphane, a substance discovered in cruciferous vegetables like broccoli and kale, has been shown to dramatically protect laboratory animals from cancer. Certain fatty acids present in fish and flaxseed protect against inflammation.

Nutraceuticals need to be looked at for precisely what they can do in the body. Let's set aside the classic divisions and definitions and examine how these nutrients can help us now, today.

MY APPROACH TO NUTRITION

Study after study shows that disease is clearly linked to low levels of nutrients. These low levels may be due to improper or deficient diets. They may also be due to the stress of fighting off illness, stress that requires greater than normal stores of important vitamins and minerals. We don't have all the answers yet.

What we do know—and what I see in my practice every day—is that when patients flood their bodies with properly monitored levels of special nutrients targeted to treat asthma, they regain their health. The nutrients I recommend fall into the following general categories:

1. Nutrients that treat underlying inflammation
2. Nutrients that encourage bronchodilation
3. Nutrients that serve as antihistamines
4. Nutrients that help the body clean up and repair damaged tissue

Some nutrients are so useful in treating asthma that they seem to have more than one effect. Others are targeted specifically to one of the four groups above.

What follows is a thumbnail sketch of the nutrients that

I find most useful in treating asthma. No patient takes every single one of these nutrients: a protocol is tailored to specific symptoms. A patient with seasonal allergies, like Rita, a thirty-two-year-old illustrator and mother of two, needs an herb called stinging nettles every spring and summer. Another patient, like Joseph, a thirty-nine-year-old diabetic with food allergies, needs nutrients like glutamine and omega-3 fatty acids to calm inflammation in the digestive tract.

What I offer first, then, is a basic nutrient protocol that can be used by any asthmatic. In order to devise a complete, full-range nutrient program, you must work with a physician who is skilled and knowledgeable about nutrition. You can use your CAP questionnaire and personal history to determine where your problem areas might be, but I recommend that you then work with your doctor in hand-tailoring a nutrient protocol.

THE BASIC ASTHMA PROTOCOL

Magnesium. If I had to recommend one nutrient to asthmatics, it would be magnesium. Over half a century ago, scientists reported that magnesium sulfate worked as a natural bronchodilator, one that opened constricted bronchial tubes without side effects. Though magnesium alone cannot cure a severe attack, intravenous magnesium sulfate is now used at many hospitals along with drugs to treat attacks. Magnesium helps relax smooth muscle, rapidly opens the bronchial tubes, and as at least one report has shown, can prevent intubation (a painful procedure in which a tube is forced down the throat to help a patient breathe).

Magnesium works at a cellular level, most likely by displacing calcium. Calcium stimulates one of the primary allergic cells in the body—the mast cell—to burst and release a flood of histamine. It is also necessary for muscle contraction. Magnesium, in contrast, helps stabilize the mast cell and relax muscles, so it functions as both an anti-inflammatory nutrient and as a bronchodilator.

Only a hospital or a trained physician can administer intravenous magnesium. I find that intravenous magnesium, along with other nutrients such as vitamin C and the B vitamins, can be extraordinarily helpful to my patients. Intravenous infusions of nutrients at levels shown to be safe can go straight into the cell in a matter of minutes. An oral supplement must be broken down and digested before it can be absorbed, and that process can be derailed by faulty enzymes or low levels of hydrochloric acid in the stomach. Therefore, oral supplements are not always sufficient, especially in patients who suffer from digestive problems.

One forty-year-old male executive who came to me was extremely skeptical about IVs. He felt so much better the day after his first IV that he returned religiously for a treatment every week for the next ten weeks. Now he is on a maintenance regimen of one IV every two months.

I find intravenous infusions to be most helpful at the beginning of a treatment program, when I want to replenish long-depleted levels of nutrients. Finally, intravenous magnesium is useful for acute attacks of asthma.

Supplements of oral magnesium can be useful over the long term. I recommend daily oral supplementation to all asthmatics. My preference is a combination of magnesium aspartate, orotate, and glycinate, in a dose of 500 milligrams a day. (As mentioned in chapter 4, accurate magnesium levels can only be obtained through an RBC magnesium test. Standard blood tests only tell you how much free magnesium is floating in the blood, and studies have shown that blood levels can be normal while cells themselves are deficient.) A note of caution: excess oral magnesium can cause diarrhea and lead to hypermagnesemia.

Antiinflammatories

Omega-3 fatty acids. Another star in the nutritional arsenal, omega-3 fatty acids are found in flaxseed and fish oils and are particularly high in fatty, deep-water fish like salmon, tuna, and mackerel. Actually incorporating itself into the fatty membrane that surrounds a cell, fish oil works as a natural antiinflammatory substance that inhibits a powerful, hormone-like substance known as prostaglandin E_2.

In general, oils such as omega-3 fatty acids are beneficial for the body. Other oils, such as omega-6 fatty acids, are important but can lead to inflammation when taken in excess. Omega-6 fatty acids have been linked to cancer in studies at the Strang Institute in New York City. They do not necessarily cause cancer, but they increase the activity of carcinogenic end-products of estrogen.

Studies on fish oil have produced uneven results, mainly because the length of the studies has varied enormously, from ten weeks to a year. Most studies have shown a significant response at the cellular level within ten weeks, so that key inflammatory cells (called neutrophils) quiet down and fire significantly fewer red-alert messages.

More important, fish oils moderate the late-phase reaction. Asthma involves both an acute inflammatory response and a secondary, late-phase reaction that can occur up to twenty-four hours later and last for weeks. That late-phase response is now believed to be the cause of chronic asthma and tissue damage, and it is halted by fish oils. A dramatic clinical response, however, can take as long as six to nine months. That seems to be how long it takes to repair long-term damage to the lungs. Remember, unlike drugs, fish oils offer a gentle treatment that slowly, over time, helps the body repair tissue damage.

One caveat: studies have shown that for asthmatics who are sensitive to aspirin, fish oils may actually intensify asthma. About 10 percent of asthmatics who are aspirin sensitive did not respond to fish oil or found that the nutrient intensified their asthma. Aspirin sensitivity is most often found in patients who suffer from asthma and nasal polyps. In addition, high levels of fish oils can thin the blood. This can be beneficial for those at risk for heart disease. It can also be a problem for asthmatics at risk for strokes. Before you take fish oils, check with your doctor to be sure that your circulatory and cardiac systems are in good shape.

For those who cannot eat fish—either because they are vegetarians, do not like the taste of fish, or are allergic to fish—another option is flaxseed oil, which contains omega-3 fatty acids. I treated one nine-year-old asthmatic who couldn't stand the fish oil capsules because she belched up a fish taste after swallowing them. Flaxseed was a reasonable substitute for her.

Fish oils can be the key nutrient for some asthmatics. One patient of mine, a forty-nine-year-old mother, went in for cosmetic surgery recently. She had been taking fish oils for a year and had been off cortisone during that time. Because fish oils can thin the blood and increase bleeding, she went off them before surgery and did not take them during the eight weeks required for total healing to the head, neck, and face. She began to notice her symptoms returning during that period and had to resume supplements for a month before she felt fine again.

I generally recommend 6 grams (6 capsules) of fish oil a day to patients who regularly eat fish, and up to 12 capsules a day for those who are not fish eaters. For strict vegetarians, enough omega-3 fatty acids can be obtained from 3 tablespoons of flaxseed oil a day. Both magnesium and fish oils help slow the inflammatory response.

Borage oil and evening primrose oil. Both these oils, obtained from plants and seeds, provide vegetable sources of GLA, gamma linoleic acid. Borage oil has about four times as much GLA as does primrose oil. GLA is an important fatty acid that some of us have a hard time making because we lack sufficient enzymes.

Another important function of GLA is that the body can transform it into omega-3 fatty acids, although we need sufficient enzymes in our body to do so. The enzyme that is used to transform GLA into omega-3 is also necessary to create inflammatory chemicals from other plant oils. Therefore, by supplementing GLA, you can use up the enzyme in creating "good" oils and reduce inflammation. Our bodies prefer omega-3 oils to all other oils, and our cells absorb them rapidly. There are a few supplements available that offer both omega-3's from fish oils, and GLA from plant oils. That, in my opinion, is an excellent combination. I recommend 3 grams of borage or primrose oil a day, in three divided doses.

Feverfew. Known officially as tanacetum parthenium, feverfew first became famous for its proven ability to treat migraines. It is rich in two powerful plant chemicals known as parthenolide and sesquiterpenes. A double-blind study published in a prominent British medical journal found that 50 milligrams daily of freeze-dried feverfew significantly reduced migraine headaches in seventeen patients. Another double-blind study of sixty migraine patients confirmed these results. Feverfew seems to inhibit inflammatory chemicals known as prostaglandins as well as histamine. It has also been shown to inhibit bacteria and yeasts. I recommend 750 milligrams a day in two divided doses.

PAF inhibitors. Platelet-activating-factor inhibitors are an exciting new avenue of treatment. Platelets are blood cells that perform a wide variety of functions. They cause blood to clot. They are also part of the inflammatory cascade. (Both inflammation and clotting are important for wound healing.) However, because PAF is part of the inflammatory cascade, it can be a potent trigger of allergies. By dampening levels of PAF, allergies and asthma may be eased. Used in conjunction with fish oils, PAF fighters can help down-regulate the inflammatory arm of the immune system. (Feverfew, for instance, contains one ingredient, parthenolide, that inhibits PAF.) I currently use two other PAF fighters, ginkgo and alkylglycerol.

Ginkgo. One of the most famous Chinese herbs, ginkgo is taken from a tree fabled to ensure long life and has long been prescribed for allergies in traditional Chinese medicine. It is now being studied in America for use in Alzheimer's disease, because it increases circulation (including blood flow to the brain). Ginkgo contains potent chemicals such as flavonglycosides, proanthocyanadins, and terpenes. Most important, animal studies show that ginkgo reduces circulating PAF and may help prevent allergic asthma.

Ginkgo should be taken as a standardized extract of 24 percent, at 40 milligrams a tablet or capsule. I recommend 3 tablets a day, in three divided doses.

Alkylglycerol. An extract of shark oil, this supplement contains alcohol ethers by that name. These fats are present in high concentrations in bone marrow, the spleen, and the liver and have been shown to stimulate the immune system and inhibit tumor growth. These alcohol ethers dampen the PAF response. I recommend 1 or 2 capsules three times a day.

Bronchodilators

In addition to magnesium, there are a few potent herbs that can open up bronchial tubes. However, I recommend that you take these herbs only under the supervision of a knowledgeable physician and/or herbalist who is working with your physician. Simply taking herbs randomly can be dangerous. A recent patient of mine was suffering from toxic levels of theophylline because of a Chinese herbal formula that had been mixed up for her by an herbalist. She was taking the herbal formula every hour, and because the formula contained high doses of theophylline, she was actually suffering from toxic blood levels. You can imagine her surprise, for she had turned to herbs in order to avoid "drugs"!

It isn't often that I see a case like that, but it does indicate a need for caution and supervision. I recommend herbs because, in general, they are gentler than drugs and often contain many active ingredients that work synergistically to improve health.

Ma huang. This herb is cultivated in China and has been used for centuries as an herbal remedy. It contains ephedrine, the chemical used in much greater amounts in asthma medications like Tedral. Ephedrine is a nervous system stimulant. Ma huang can reduce swelling in the mucous lining of nasal passages and sinuses. It is a potent bronchodilator. I like to use it for cough associated with asthma because of the soothing effect of the warm tea as it is swallowed and because the ephedra can go right into the mucous membranes. This herb can be found in most health food stores and in herbal tea formulas for asthma. This should not be used by individuals with high blood pressure or heart disease.

Cayenne. Capsicum, or red pepper, stimulates secretion of saliva and thins mucus plugs. It is a stimulant that warms the body, and its active ingredient, capsaicin, has been shown to desensitize the airways of rats to irritants. It reduces the edema and permeability caused by respiratory irritants. This should be used with caution by individuals with peptic ulcer disease.

As you will see, I recommend liberal use of cayenne in cooking. Some patients do well on cayenne, but patients in an acute state of illness may find that it aggravates their intestinal tract. For those who enjoy the taste and warmth of cayenne, I recommend up to 1,000 milligrams a day in three divided doses and/or liberal use in foods.

Coleus forskholii. This herb has been used for centuries in Indian Ayurvedic medicine. It is a rich source of biologically active compounds. The active ingredient, forskolin, helps increase compounds in the body that relax bronchial muscle. Several double-blind studies have shown that the herb is as effective as the drug fenoterol, without the side effects of shakiness and tremors. Standardized extracts of the herb are most effective if they contain 18 percent forskolin. I recommend 50 milligrams two or three times a day.

Turmeric and ginger. Turmeric is a perennial herb of the ginger family used in Chinese medicine as an antiinflammatory agent. Its active ingredient is curcumin. Ginger, in turn, is native to Southeast Asia. It is known as a warming remedy in traditional Chinese medicine and so is considered useful in colds. Ginger is a potent inhibitor of prostaglandins, inflammatory chemicals. I prefer ginger in herbal tinctures and teas. Fresh ginger can be sliced, simmered for about twenty minutes in water, and sweetened with honey or milk.

Licorice. This is an extensively studied herb whose formal name is glycyrrhiza glabra. It contains antiallergic, antibacterial, and antiinflammatory compounds. Two of its components have cortisol-like effects in the body. One ingredient in licorice can raise blood pressure, but deglycyrrhizinated commercial products eliminate this problem. Such a product, DGL, is available as a powder, tablet, or tincture. Twenty to 40 drops of a tincture in very hot water can be taken as a tea, three times a day. Licorice in its pure form is the preferred treatment, however.

Compound Herbal Elixir. This product, produced by Eclectic Institute, is used widely by naturopaths and physicians around the country. It is recommended for cough and asthma and contains a wide range of ingredients, including wildcrafted wild cherry, organic elecampane, red clover blossoms, lobelia, fennel, lomatium dissectum, white pine, and essential oil of bitter orange. These ingredients work together to stimulate the immune system, treat the symptoms of asthma, and purify the lymph and bloodstream.

Antihistamines

Vitamin C. This vitamin works as a gentle antihistamine without the side effects of medications. It is also a superstar vitamin that serves as an antioxidant. I recommend 3 grams (3,000 milligrams) a day, in three divided doses.

Stinging nettles. This herb has been utilized for decades as a medicinal agent and edible plant. However, the stinging hairs of fresh nettle leaves contain histamine as well as chemicals that actually liberate histamine when you eat the plant. We don't know why, but somehow this histamine seems to help allergic people. It sounds paradoxical, but in a double-blind study of sixty-nine individuals with allergic rhinitis, nearly 50 percent found stinging nettles as effective as their regular medications.

I use nettles for asthma patients with sinus problems or nasal allergies. Care must be taken to obtain a good brand of nettles that has been properly harvested in the spring, when the potent constituents of the stinging leaves are present. I generally recommend 2 capsules, three times a day.

Quercetin. This is a potent bioflavonoid that has been well documented for its antiallergic and antihistamine properties. I find it very helpful for allergies and recommend 300 milligrams a day in three divided doses.

Histidine. This amino acid is actually a building block for histamine. For reasons not fully understood, supplements of histidine seem to reduce allergic symptoms. I recommend 1,500 milligrams in three divided doses daily.

Star Nutrients

Vitamins C and E and beta-carotene. This famous triumvirate of free-radical quenchers is being widely studied. In fact, the National Institutes of Health (NIH) now has over a dozen studies under way on beta-carotene and cancer. Each of these nutrients works in a special way.

Vitamin E is a fat-soluble nutrient that penetrates each cell's fatty membrane and, once there, protects the cell from damage. It is especially good at neutralizing rancid fats that have themselves been damaged by free radicals. In particular, vitamin E neutralizes the damaging effects of ozone, a major component of smog. Since studies have shown that asthma and allergies worsen in general after exposure to ozone, this is a necessary nutrient for asthmatics. I recommend 400 international units a day of vitamin E.

Vitamin C deactivates free radicals and stimulates white blood cells to fight infection. It has been proven to directly kill many bacteria and viruses, and finally, it has the ability to recycle vitamin E. After vitamin E has neutralized a free radical, it becomes inactive. In the presence of vitamin C, it can become active again. I recommend 3 grams a day, in three divided doses. Vitamin C can be obtained in a buffered or esterized form so that it does not cause diarrhea and is more easily absorbed.

Beta-carotene and other carotenoids are potent free-radical quenchers. Low carotene levels are linked with decreased white blood counts and decreased ability of the white blood cells to fight infection. Low levels have also been linked with an increased incidence of lung cancer. There are over six hundred forms of carotene found in natural sources, but only 10 percent can serve as building blocks for vitamin A. Those 10 percent, including beta-carotene, can be converted by the body into vitamin A, which is crucial for healthy lung tissue. I recommend up to 25,000 international units a day.

B vitamins. All the B vitamins are crucial for energy production in the body. Vitamins B_5, B_6, and B_{12} are particularly helpful.

Vitamin B_5, or pantothenic acid, is a building block for cortisone. When B_5 is deficient the adrenal glands become weak and compromised. Allergies are often a sign of B_5 deficiency. B_5 has been shown to enhance production of adrenal hormones, sometimes in as little as twenty-four hours.

Vitamin B_6 is involved in more bodily functions than any other nutrient. Studies have shown that B_6 can improve asthma. Asthmatics with very low levels of B_6 in its active, usable form improved dramatically when given 50 milligrams of the vitamin twice a day.

Vitamin B_{12} boosts energy and immunity and is especially helpful in combating fatigue associated with chronic illness.

Though individual needs for B vitamins vary widely, my basic daily recommendation for moderate to severe asthma is 50 milligrams of B_2 and B_3, 100 milligrams of B_1, 500 milligrams of B_5, 150 milligrams of B_6, 1,000 micrograms of B_{12}. These vitamins are water soluble, so excess amounts are quickly excreted in the urine. Divided doses enhance absorption.

Zinc. Low levels of zinc, an important mineral for immunity, have been linked to poor wound healing and frequent infections, as well as loss of taste. Moderate zinc deficiency is associated with impaired ability to react to specific antigens, such as allergens, while severe deficiency is linked with recurrent infection. (On the other hand, excess zinc can sometimes cause problems, particularly in Alzheimer's patients.) High doses of zinc (over 100 milligrams a day) for longer than a month can displace other minerals, including copper and iron. Therefore, I recommend 50 milligrams a day. For long-term use over 3 months, I recommend 25 milligrams daily.

Vitamin A. An important element in the treatment of asthma, vitamin A ensures the health of mucus-producing epithelial tissue in the lining of the mouth, nose, and lungs. Those low in vitamin A are more susceptible to upper respiratory infections. This vitamin is fat soluble and is stored in the tissues and liver, so it needs to be given in judicious amounts. Excess vitamin A can be toxic. I do recommend supplements, however. Many people forgo vitamin A entirely, taking its precursor, beta-carotene. They do not realize that beta-carotene is useful in its original form as an antioxidant and that the body uses energy to convert beta-carotene to vitamin A. Therefore, modest supplementation with vitamin A, about 5,000 international units daily, is something I recommend. More than 5,000 units a day can be dangerous, especially in women of childbearing years.

Ginseng. Formally known as eleuthroccocus senticosus, ginseng root is a member of a class of herbs called adaptogens, herbs that normalize the metabolism, whether it is overactive or underactive. Ginseng has been found to help those with hypertension as well as hypotension, for instance. It is very helpful in treating fatigue and low energy. The root contains sterols, coumarins, lignans, and other compounds that seem to increase energy and the ability to tolerate stress. Ginseng extracts vary widely according to the company that manufactures them, but I recommend 800 milligrams a day in capsule form in two divided doses.

Echinacea. One of the most studied herbs in the world, echinacea (purple coneflower) is antiinfective, antibacterial, and antiviral. The herb stimulates our immune system's B-cells and T-cells, as well as interferon. It aids in tissue regeneration and is excellent as a general immune booster. According to Ed Alstat, a pharmacist and founder of Eclectic Institute, it is the long-chain sugars, or mucopolysaccharides, that are responsible for echinacea's immune-boosting capacity. Those complex sugars are also present in other herbs, says Alstat, and he has extracted them in a formula known as Atomic Echinacea. In addition, notes Alstat, tinctures of echinacea often leach out these beneficial long-chain sugars. Freeze-dried herbs preserve the plant better. I recommend about 800 milligrams a day in two divided doses.

Shiitake mushrooms. Known as lentinus edodes, shiitake mushrooms—along with other mushrooms now being studied, such as reishi and maitake—are immune stimulants. They also contain complex polysaccharides that boost T-cells and interferon. Raw or cooked, mushrooms are recommended in any diet. Capsules of freeze-dried mushroom extracts can also be of benefit. I recommend 800 milligrams a day in two divided doses.

N-acetylcysteine (NAC). This amino acid is a free-radical scavenger. It potentiates the body's use of vitamin C. It is also a building block for glutathione, one of the most powerful free-radical quenchers available to the body. Glutathione helps the liver detoxify medications, histamine, and other harmful substances. Finally, NAC has been used therapeutically to reduce mucus buildup. I recommend 500 milligrams twice a day.

Selenium. One of the ten essential trace minerals, selenium is another vital building block for glutathione, and it also helps vitamin E quench free radicals. Selenium is also an antioxidant and helps maintain the integrity of cell membranes, protecting against toxins and toxic metals. I generally recommend 200 micrograms a day.

Garlic. For over four thousand years, the Chinese have maintained that garlic has a wide range of benefits, from battling infection to helping prevent heart disease and cancer. Though garlic is not a cure-all, recent research has confirmed that garlic's sulfur-containing compounds do have active pharmacological activity. The amounts vary from variety to variety, and even from bulb to bulb, but garlic's saponins (steroidlike compounds) reduce blood pressure, reduce the stickiness of blood platelets better than aspirin, reduce the risk of colon and stomach cancer, and slow deterioration of the brain. In animal studies, one garlic compound, diallyl disulfide, was found to be very effective in inhibiting tumor growth. I recommend liberal use of garlic or, if you dislike the odor, odorless garlic capsules or oil. However, these may lack some of the beneficial compounds.

As this book goes to press, our knowledge of the benefits of natural therapies continues to grow. In a letter to the *New York Times* in June of 1996, Mark Blumenthal, executive director of the American Botanical Council, noted that "Thousands of studies are conducted each year on the chemistry, pharmacology, toxicology, and clinical use of hundreds of herbs, their individual chemical constituents and whole extracts containing numerous compounds." Another letter by David Eisenberg, M.D., director of the Center of Alternative Medicine Research at Beth Israel Hospital/Harvard Medical School, concluded, "There is a Chinese proverb: 'Real gold is not afraid of the hottest fire.' It is the responsibility of the medical establishment to ensure that these therapies do not remain untested forever."

A MAINTENANCE PROTOCOL

As I have mentioned, I don't recommend all of the above to any individual patient. The above nutrients are my basic nutritional arsenal. However, I do recommend that all asthma patients take a blend of basic vitamins and minerals. A daily maintenance program should include 1,000 milligrams of vitamin C; 10,000 international units of beta-carotene; 400 international units of vitamin E; and 500 milligrams of magnesium.

IN CONCLUSION

I'd like to return for a moment to the efficacy of intravenous supplements. Hospital studies have shown that IV magnesium is beneficial. I find that in acute asthma, IV vitamins including a formulation of preservative-free vitamin C, magnesium, and B vitamins, can be tremendously helpful. They drip directly into the vein and are instantly available for use by the body. Most of my patients who begin with IVs stabilize quickly, needing them later only in times of extreme stress or for a flare-up. Before and after surgery or air travel, for instance, IVs can help protect asthmatics from a relapse.

As for Kris, her health improved so rapidly after embarking on a treatment program that she took a modeling assignment in Europe. Another patient, George, was suffering so badly from allergies and asthma that his wife was ready to divorce him. He was allergic to so many substances that he was unable to concentrate at work or sleep through the night.

"If I even touched a dog or cat, I'd have a terrible reaction," George recalled. "If I petted a dog once and didn't wash my hands, my eyes were red within five seconds and I was sneezing. Everybody in the office knew me as the guy who walked around with a box of Kleenex. They joked that I must be a cocaine addict."

After a protocol of magnesium, vitamin C, B vitamins, ginseng, stinging nettles, and fish oils, he improved quickly.

"I have never had a year like this," George said. "Before, I couldn't go to bed at night without medication. After two months on your program, I can sleep through the night without drugs. But if I stop my vitamin therapy for a few weeks, my symptoms return, the asthma, bronchitis, the whole thing. I tried that in January, and I was a mess, hacking and coughing. So now I'm religious about my vitamins and my monthly IVs. I don't want to suffer again!"

A nurse who works in hospital admissions came to me after she was hospitalized for the third time in a year for acute asthma. A year later, after an intensive vitamin protocol in the context of the CAP program, she has had no severe attacks.

"I just ran my first road race," one of my patients, Trish, a thirty-four-year-old producer, recently told me. When she first came to my office, she was taking daily doses of prednisone, theophylline, and Ventolin. She was fatigued and depressed. Her "medications" now are magnesium, vitamin C, fish oils, ginkgo, and IVs once a month. She uses her Ventolin inhaler on occasion. "Last year everyone said I looked pale and tired. I didn't travel. Now I'm going to Paris next week—for the pure fun of it."

As more information about the benefits of nutrients unfolds, we will be able to refine the protocols we create to combat illness. Nutritional medicine is, I believe, the direction we will turn to in the future. We now understand that it isn't just a few nutrients, but a broad family of powerful substances in our foods, that can prevent illness. Hopefully, in the coming years more research will be done in this area.

That brings me to the next piece of my program: foods themselves. Foods themselves can be your best medicine: by eliminating foods that harm, and emphasizing foods that heal, you can go a long way toward preserving health.

DOCTOR'S RECOMMENDATIONS FOR ACTION

1. Nutritional deficiencies are an important cause of chronic asthma. Nutrient supplementation targets asthma at a cellular level and can be surprisingly effective. Many nutrients and herbs have been proven in studies to be helpful in treating the symptoms of chronic illnesses such as asthma.

2. Think of nutrients as nutraceuticals—compounds in our foods that can be used to help heal us. Although we have created classes of nutrients, such as vitamins and minerals,

that concept is actually simplistic. Vitamins, for instance, can act like hormones in some cases. Fatty acids present in fish can protect against inflammation. Compounds in broccoli can fight cancer.

3. Make sure you are taking nutraceuticals that fall into all four categories needed for healing: nutrients that treat inflammation, that encourage bronchodilation, that work like antihistamines, and that help the body repair damaged tissue.

4. Consider taking magnesium, orally or (if blood tests indicate it is necessary) intravenously. Studies have shown that magnesium works as a natural bronchodilator. I consider it an essential nutrient in asthma.

5. Make sure your diet contains enough omega-3 fatty acids, found in flaxseed and fish oils, as well as deep-water fish like salmon, tuna, and mackerel. Fish oil works as a natural antiinflammatory substance, and studies show that over a period of months, it can significantly reduce inflammation. Remember, it's the ratio of omega-3 oils to omega-6 oils that is important.

6. If you are taking fish oil supplements, be sure to take vitamin E at the same time. Any oil can oxidize, causing free-radical damage. Vitamin E can prevent this.

7. Talk to your physician about taking herbs such as feverfew and ginkgo, both of which are antiinflammatory. Consider other supplements such as nettles, ma huang, cayenne, licorice, echinacea, or herbal asthma formulas. All can be effective in treating symptoms of allergies and asthma. Although many herbs have not been standardized, there is a mounting body of evidence to support their beneficial effects.

8. At the very least, take a general asthma protocol of nutrients, which includes vitamin C, vitamin A, vitamin E, zinc, magnesium, B complex, and beta-carotene.

9. I have developed specific supplements for all nutrients mentioned in this chapter. For more information call Nutriceutical Research, Inc. (NRI) at 1-800-ANTI-OX-ABC.

CHAPTER EIGHT

Foods That Harm and Foods That Heal

It's nearly impossible for me to sing the praises of nutrients without—in the very same breath—speaking of food. In the last few years, vitamins, minerals, and "celebrity" nutrients like beta-carotene have moved to center stage. Millions of health-conscious Americans daily take supplements in the hopes of staving off illness and aging. A veritable avalanche of laboratory studies indicates that antioxidant nutrients may indeed help protect against damage from oxidation and free radicals.

Yet no cornucopia of nutrients, no matter how rich and varied, can substitute for the healing power of a good, healthful diet. This cannot be emphasized enough where asthma is concerned. A 1996 conference of the American Lung Association and the American Thoracic Society in New Orleans presented truly remarkable evidence of the link between diet and asthma. Australian researchers found that a healthy diet actually *prevents* asthma symptoms in children. A good diet early in life may actually prevent a lifetime of chronic illness! The researchers found specifically that fat and sugar are linked to asthma attacks, and children with a higher intake of fish and fish oils had fewer asthma symptoms. Another study published in *Thorax* in 1997 confirmed that diet plays a crucial role in the development of Asthma. In the late 1980s, the average American ate about 1½ servings of vegetables a day, less than a single serving of fruit, and less than one-third of one serving of beans or nuts—and those servings are tiny: about half a cup. Researchers are now recommending at least five servings a day of fruits and vegetables, as well as generous portions of healthy legumes like beans and nuts. Some studies involve individuals eating eight servings of fruits and vegetables a day. If this is a stretch for you, try to eat as many servings as you comfortably can.

The latest research finds that plants are literally loaded with thousands of powerful phytochemicals that may work in countless, still mysterious ways to keep us healthy. Certain families of foods, such as cruciferous vegetables (broccoli, brussels sprouts, cabbage) are particularly rich in compounds that may prevent cancer. Onions and garlic have proven quite potent against infection and disease in certain experiments. From flavones in beans, to indoles in broccoli, to genistein in soybeans, phytochemicals may just be the "magic bullets" of the future.

HEALING PLANTS

Phytochemicals protect plant cells from toxins, and they go right on doing the same job in our cells when we consume vegetables and fruits. Here's a sampling of recent findings from laboratory research:

- Limonen in citrus fruits boosts production of enzymes that help neutralize potential carcinogens.
- Allyl sulfides in garlic, onions, leeks, and chives stimulate levels of glutathione S-transferase, one of the primary detoxification enzymes.
- Dithiolthiones in broccoli boost levels of enzymes that stop carcinogens from damaging cells.
- Ellagic acid in grapes and strawberries neutralizes free radicals.

- Isoflavones in soybeans block the absorption of estrogen by cells, thus reducing the risk of certain estrogen-dependent malignancies such as breast cancer. Other flavonoids in fruits and vegetables, from carrots to berries, block receptor sites for hormones that may promote cancer.
- Genistein is a compound found in high concentrations in soybeans and in cruciferous vegetables such as broccoli and cabbage. In laboratory test-tube experiments, it was found that genistein blocks angiogenesis, the growth of new blood vessels. Angiogenesis can be necessary, for example, in a heart patient when his or her body forms alternate routes of blood flow. But in certain diseases, such as cancer, it can allow the tumor to spread and grow.
- Monoterpenes—found in parsley, carrots, yams, tomatoes, eggplants, basil, citrus fruits, broccoli, and other vegetables—are antioxidants. They also boost immunoprotective enzymes.

For the past two decades, researchers around the world have consistently made the same discovery: those individuals who eat large amounts of vegetables and fruits have lower rates of most cancers. A study in the journal *Nutrition and Cancer* reviewed 156 separate studies on fruits, vegetables, and cancer risk and found that people who eat a diet high in fruits and vegetables have about half the normal risk of developing most cancers. The author of the study, Gladys Block, professor of public health at the University of California at Berkeley, recommends five servings of fruits and vegetables a day. She announced, "There are some cancers for which one nutrient is more important than another. But then the opposite is true for another cancer. Nature packaged them all together in fruits and vegetables."

Even so, nutrition is still regarded with suspicion by many otherwise brilliant, mainstream researchers. They are wary of the so-called hype surrounding nutritional claims, and thus studies about nutrition and health are still in their infancy.

"It's all well and good to say eat more vegetables," Dr. Paul Talalay of Johns Hopkins School of Medicine told *The New York Times* last year. "But the data are extraordinarily soft on what we mean by that. We're trying to survey all these vegetables . . . and it's extremely slow going."

The day may come when we can genetically engineer superfoods that contain high concentrations of healing nutrients whose specific effects we have studied and quantified in laboratories.

Until that day, how can you take the newest findings about nutrition and apply it to your own life as an asthmatic? As an asthma sufferer myself and as a physician who has treated asthmatics, I have found that certain foods can have significant benefits. They can truly help ameliorate asthma. I see it every day in my practice. As reported at an international conference on asthma in 1996 in New Orleans, we are now beginning to understand links between asthma and diet that are similar in importance to research fifteen years ago that linked saturated fat to heart disease.

At the same time, foods can cause significant health problems, especially for the allergic patient. Many of my asthma patients turn out to be highly sensitive to foods they eat daily. Those foods can set off immune reactions that simply raise their levels of allergic antibodies and intensify allergic inflammation. That sets the stage for an asthma attack.

Aside from food sensitivities, certain foods are known to promote inflammation. In particular, animal meats, animal fats, and partially hydrogenated fats lead to greater levels of inflammatory prostaglandins (prostaglandins, you will remember, are powerful, hormone-like chemicals). Other compounds—such as sulfites—can lead directly to asthma attacks in sensitive individuals. Histamine in wine, strawberries, and other foods may intensify allergies and asthma.

Take Pat, a forty-five-year-old tennis professional and asthmatic. She finds that if she is not absolutely careful about staying on a specific diet (which I nickname the Park Avenue Spa diet), her asthma returns and her tennis game is severely impaired. At a recent tennis tournament, she came down with a bronchial infection that ruined her game. "I'd been eating the wrong foods," she admitted somewhat sheepishly.

Yes, foods can harm you. That's the bad news. The good news is that many foods are powerful healers for the condition of asthma. Fish, which contains omega-3 oils, eases inflammation. Bioflavonoids in citrus fruits, pineapples, and other foods can prevent histamine release. Mushrooms, mentioned in the last chapter, boost the immune system. Carrots contain beta-carotene, an antioxidant. Tomatoes contain an equally strong carotenoid. Foods have many healing properties.

MY APPROACH TO DIET

I consider the following elements in crafting healthy diets:

1. Food allergies and sensitivities
2. Foods that may exacerbate asthma and inflammation in general
3. Foods that quench inflammation and free radicals or open bronchial tubes
4. Healthy cooking that requires no recipes, requires minimal cooking time, and can be easily learned and adapted so that a healthy diet is easy to achieve
5. An overview of what is healthy in supermarket foods and restaurant meals so that patients learn healthy shopping and healthy dining

YOUR DIET REVOLUTION:
FROM HARMFUL TO HELPFUL

It sounds simple, doesn't it? Adopt a healthful diet, and not only will your asthma improve, but you will also be protecting your well-being and nourishing yourself with healing substances.

Yet food is never a simple matter. Eating, as we all know, can be symbolic of love (have you ever cooked a meal for a new flame in the first flush of romance?), hate (have you ever stuffed down a bag of munchies when you were angry at someone?), or social acceptance (consider the crudités offered at parties). It can be a substitute for nurturing (ice cream on a lonely Saturday night); a way of "swallowing" and "stuffing" feelings (eating when you're sad or anxious); a pleasant habit indulged in out of boredom (snacking at home when there's nothing else to do). Unhealthy foods— from hamburgers to pastries, sugary breakfast cereals, candy bars, and ice cream—leap out at us from every restaurant window, from advertising pages of magazines and newspapers, and on television commercials.

Most of us have food lapses from time to time, where we cannot resist biting into that sumptuous bar of gourmet chocolate or that gleaming wedge of fresh cheesecake. Few of us can—or have to—maintain absolutely perfect, pristine diets 100 percent of the time. On the other hand, I've gone to the homes of friends who claim they follow a healthy diet, opened their refrigerators, and found so-called "health" cookies, crackers, milk products, cheese spreads, sodas, margarine, doughnuts, ice cream, salted crackers, and a treasure chest of other unhealthy foods.

I nicknamed one of my asthmatic friends the Condiment King because his refrigerator was filled with ketchup, relish, barbecue sauce, and literally dozens of bottles of garnishes and condiments. His freezer, in turn, was stacked with hamburger buns. In the summer, he grilled hamburgers in his backyard nearly every day, spraying himself with a good dose from his inhaler before he played catch with his kids.

A FRESH START: FIND OUT ABOUT FOOD ALLERGIES

Remember Kris, who in the last chapter told how she suffered her first terrifying asthma attack while on a ski vacation with her family? She happened to be suffering from a few severe food allergies, which showed up on scratch tests: apples, strawberries, wheat, and eggs. These foods were some of her favorites: she ate a lot of pizza during her busy days modeling and always carried a snack of apples and hard-boiled eggs in her backpack. Here's her story in her own words:

> I thought eggs and apples were healthy, a balanced protein and natural fruit, and they were so convenient. I also figured that pizza topped with vegetables was a better food than hamburgers or hot dogs. I couldn't believe it when I found out I was allergic to eggs, wheat, and cheese. But a friend of mine with allergies had gone to you and you'd done wonders for her, so I decided I'd do what you suggested.
>
> I changed my diet and added vitamins and minerals, and it worked so quickly. Within two weeks I felt great. I could walk down the street and go up and down the subway stairs ten times a day without feeling out of breath. I used to have to catch my breath every time I walked up stairs. Now I'm not waking up at night, either. I'm sleeping well. I feel really good now. But I have to confess that I do cheat on my diet sometimes and eat what I'm not supposed to.

Not all my patients suffer from food allergies, but many do. Often they have no clue about their allergies. I had a patient who, discussing her diet, said, "Maybe it's the yogurt in the morning? The chocolate bar I have in the afternoon? What do you think?" When I examined a food diary, I found that she was eating peanuts three or four times a day.

How do you determine if you suffer from food allergies or food sensitivities? First, you need a clear definition of food allergy. Because food allergy is a controversial concept in some circles—especially among mainstream allergists—I prefer to speak of adverse responses to foods. Adverse responses can include: anaphylactic, allergic, and delayed allergic reactions.

Anaphylactic reactions to food occur instantly and can be so severe that they end in death. Anaphylactic reactions may include swelling of the lips, tongue, and throat, acute exacerbation of asthma, dizziness, difficulty breathing, anxiety, vomiting, diarrhea. One tragic instance of a fatal anaphylactic reaction was a student at Brown University who knew she was allergic to peanuts and so avoided them religiously. However, one night she ordered chili at a restaurant, not knowing the chili recipe included peanut butter. She died.

Anaphylactic reactions are most frequently caused by peanuts, nuts, shellfish, eggs, and seeds. A peanut-sensitive individual may eat a peanut and be dead twenty minutes later. In fact, the medical literature is studded with truly tragic cases, where peanuts were a hidden ingredient in a food, not listed on the label, and caused the death of an unsuspecting individual.

Avoidance of anaphylactic foods is not adequate treatment for patients at risk, for they may accidentally eat the allergen-containing food. The patient must be taught to recognize when they have eaten the allergen; often a severe reaction begins with a tingling sensation on the tongue and lips. They also need to carry an emergency dose of epineph-rine—an EpiPen—and use it as soon as symptoms begin. Then they must go directly to an emergency room and stay there for several hours because of the danger of a relapse reaction after the initial reaction subsides. This kind of approach can prevent needless tragedies.

Allergic reactions to food are not as severe as anaphy-lactic reactions, and seldom fatal, but they are often imme-diate. There may be some blurring between severe allergic reactions and mild anaphylactic reactions. For instance, an allergy to sesame may cause the lips to swell and bronchial tubes to tighten, without further symptoms. Allergic reac-tions are mediated by the immunoglobulin called IgE.

Delayed allergic reactions, a more controversial con-cept, seem to be mediated by IgG, a different type of immune molecule. There are probably a cascade of inflam-matory mediators in food allergies, many of which we have not yet pinpointed. Therefore, you may find yourself fatigued or bloated hours after eating a food, or even the next day. These allergies are harder to ferret out, and they become obvious only when, after eliminating a food (or foods) from the diet, symptoms clear up. Delayed reactions can be particularly troublesome when treating children, who may eat foods at school or at friends' houses and not experience a flare-up until days or weeks later.

In some cases, an allergic response to a food may occur only at certain times—for instance, when your allergy load is high and many inflammatory chemicals are circulating in your blood. During hay fever season, for example, you may be more sensitive to specific foods, or you may suffer sensi-tivities only when multiple allergenic foods are eaten at the same time. Once your allergic load is lessened, food sensi-tivities may clear up.

Symptoms of allergies can vary. Migraine and cluster headaches are often linked to food allergies; so is a condition known as tension-fatigue syndrome, first described in 1922.

Symptoms of anxiety, irritability, nervousness, or listlessness can be triggered by food allergies. Allergies can be linked to depression, as well. Studies of depressed and chronically fatigued patients found that up to 70 percent suffered from allergies—as compared to 2 percent of healthy controls. Histamine is released in great quantities during allergic reactions.

A REVOLUTIONARY THEORY OF ALLERGY

Food allergens are most often proteins, which the body treats as antigens, or invaders. That may be because viruses and bacteria usually contain a protein coat, and our immune system learns to recognize these proteins as invaders. Foods not broken down by the digestive system may, in some cases, enter the bloodstream as undigested proteins and provoke allergic reactions.

Studies indicate that proteins in cow's milk, eggs, peanuts, wheat, and soy are the most common food allergens. Cow's milk alone contains thirty proteins that are considered antigenic to humans. Food allergies seem linked to a person's ability to properly process and break down a particular food. If a person lacks or is low in the enzymes required to break a food down to amino acids, carbohydrates, and fats, allergic symptoms may result.

Yet there is much about food allergy that still remains a mystery. Milk allergies can change over time, yet allergies to certain foods, such as peanuts, seem to last a lifetime. Sometimes an allergy to one member of a food group—such as shrimp (shellfish) or peanuts (legumes)—may lead to cross-reactivity, or allergic reactions to other members of that same food group. (See the chart beginning on page 163.) For some individuals, even inhaling steam from cooking foods can cause an allergic reaction.

Certain foods seem more provocative than others. Those

individuals who are allergic to peanuts are often sensitive to soybeans, peas, and other foods that are legumes. Yet, oddly enough, the reverse is not always true. Individuals allergic to peas or soybeans, for instance, are not necessarily allergic to peanuts. For some patients, perhaps the greatest irony in food allergy is that the foods we crave and eat the most are often the ones to which we are allergic. The mere idea of giving up those beloved foods is pure torment. Why is it that foods we eat frequently so often lead to allergies, while foods eaten on a rotation diet (no more than once every four days) are well tolerated?

I believe there is a very good reason. One theory suggests that food allergies may have started out as a protective mechanism, both for the individual and the species. Most plants contain toxins, natural pesticides, and carcinogens. Take peanuts: they tend to grow a mold called aflatoxin, a potent carcinogen that is known to cause liver damage. An allergy to peanuts may, at some time in our genetic past, have protected our forebears from being poisoned.

If we eat a food day after day, its toxins build up in our body. We develop an allergy, find the food unpleasant because of the symptoms it causes, and stop eating it for a while or, in some cases, permanently. Or we find methods of detoxifying ourselves—like the Indians in the Peruvian Andes, who eat copious amounts of clay to detoxify the potentially poisonous bitter potatoes in their diet.

Another school of thought suggests that we can also become addicted to an allergic food because our body, in response to the stress of being "challenged" with the food, releases endorphins. Endorphins are our bodies' own, natural opium-like chemicals. Perhaps endorphins ease the unpleasant allergic response, but they can fool us into thinking we need to eat the food to which we are allergic. We become addicted to the endorphin release. Only after avoiding the food for a few days or a week do we begin to lose the craving for it, along with the allergic symptoms.

ARE FOOD ALLERGIES GOOD FOR YOU?

Recently, a startling new theory about the reason for allergies has been put forth by Margie Profet, a thirty-five-year-old recipient of a MacArthur "genius" grant for her work on allergies, menstruation, and morning sickness. Profet suggests that allergies evolved as a defense against environmental toxins, which can be extremely tiny in size and so can slip through our cell membranes effortlessly.

The following process, says Profet, may explain how, after eating a peanut, a child might develop an allergy to this legume: A toxin (such as a mold) was attached to the protein in the peanut, and the immune system decides to target the protein itself. The protein is far larger and easier to attack. The symptoms of allergies—sneezing, coughing, diarrhea, vomiting, itching that makes you want to scratch—all seem to be the body's way of trying to expel a toxin.

According to Profet, we all have different genetic templates with which we are born. Because of our individual mix of genes, we have inherited different strengths and weaknesses. Some of us have greater amounts of detoxifying enzymes, which break down toxins and let us excrete them without harm. For those of us who lack enough enzymes to neutralize a particular toxin, allergy is a backup defense. By developing an allergy to the toxin, our bodies can mobilize the defenses to excrete it.

Her work takes the basic stance that the body has a reason for everything it does. Allergies are not simply a wholesale mistake on the part of nature. They may actually help protect us against some toxins.

This theory is in direct contrast to another theory, sometimes teasingly known as the "little worm theory." This theory suggests that originally IgE—the primary immune antibody—evolved to fight parasites or worms. Now that we live in a society where parasites are supposedly less common, IgE mistakenly fights other, neutral substances. There are some big questions about this theory. In addition, IgE does not seem very effective at combating parasites, since parasite infections are extremely common around the world. I personally find it hard to believe that IgE was meant to fight parasites alone, and that lacking parasites, it says to itself, "Well, I'll attack a peanut instead." Why would the body, which is typically so efficient, be so inefficient in this case?

You are probably wondering how these musings on the evolutionary significance of allergies can help you, so let me get back to how you can feel better. Understanding the way the body works is the first step in healing illness. You want to feel better. Here's how to do it.

FOOD FAMILIES

You will probably be surprised by this list of food families. Who would think that cashews and mangoes had anything in common? Or beets and spinach? Yet these foods share many common genes. Though in most cases you will not have to eliminate an entire food family because of a single allergy in that group, it's wise to pay attention to food families and to check for cross-sensitivities.

Apple Family
   Apple, crab apple, loquat, pear, quince
Arrowroot Family
   Arrowroot,
Arum Family
   Taro
Banana Family
   Banana, plantain
Barberry Family
   Barberry
Basselad Family
   Vine spinach

Beech Family
    Beechnut, chestnut
Birch Family
    Filbert, hazelnut
Borage Family
    Borage
Brazil Nut Family
    Brazil nut
Buckthorn Family
    Jujube
Buckwheat Family
    Buckwheat, rhubarb
Cactus Family
    Prickly pear
Caper Family
    Caper
Carpetweed Family
    New Zealand spinach
Cashew Family
    Cashew, mango, pistachio
Citrus Family
    Citron, grapefruit, kumquat, lemon, lime, orange,
    tangerine, tangelo
Coca Family
    Coca leaf
Cola Nut Family
    Chocolate, cola (kola) nut
Custard Apple Family
    Custard apple, pawpaw
Cycad Family
    Sago palm
Ebony Family
    Persimmon
Flax Family
    Flaxseed
Ginger Family
    Cardamom, ginger, turmeric
Ginkgo Family
    Ginkgo
Gooseberry Family
    Currant, gooseberry

Goosefoot Family
Beet, lamb's quarters, spinach, Swiss chard
Gourd Family
Cantaloupe, Casaba, Chinese watermelon, citron melon, cucumber, honeydew, muskmelon, pumpkin, squash (acorn, butternut, summer, winter), vegetable marrow, watermelon
Grape Family
American grape, European grape
Grain Family
Amaranth, bamboo, corn (maize), millet, oats, popcorn, quinoa, rice (brown, white, basmati), rye, sorghum, spelt, sugarcane, teff, wheat, wild rice
Heath Family
Blueberry, cranberry, lingonberry
Honeysuckle Family
Elderberry
Indian Plum Family
Annatto, Indian plum
Iris Family
Orris root, saffron
Laurel Family
Avocado, bay leaf, cassia, cinnamon, sassafras
Legume Family
Adzuki bean, asparagus, balsam of Peru, black-eyed pea, cowpea, broad (fava) bean, carob bean, chickpea (garbanzo), common bean (navy, kidney, pinto, string), fenugreek, guar, jack bean, lentil, licorice, lima bean, mung bean, mesquite, pea, peanut, scarlet runner bean, soybean, tamarind
Lily Family
Asparagus, chives, day lily, garlic, leek, onion, sarsaparilla, shallot
Madder Family
Black guava, coffee
Mallow Family
Cottonseed, okra
Maple Family
Maple
Mint Family
Balm, basil, bergamot, horehound, hyssop, Japanese artichoke, lavender, marjoram, oregano,

peppermint, rosemary, sage, savory, spearmint, thyme

Morning Glory Family
Sweet potato

Mulberry Family
Breadfruit, fig, hop, mulberry

Mustard Family
Arugula, broccoli, brussels sprouts, cabbage, Chinese cabbage, collards, kale, garden cress, horseradish, kohlrabi, mustard, radish, rapeseed, rutabaga, turnip, watercress, wintercress

Myrtle Family
Allspice, clove, guava, myrtle, roseapple

Nightshade Family
Bell pepper, cayenne pepper, eggplant, ground cherry, paprika, potato (white, Irish), tomato, tree tomato

Nutmeg Family
Nutmeg, mace

Olive Family
Jasmine, manna, olive

Orchid Family
Vanilla

Palm Family
Cabbage palm, coconut, date, oil palm

Papaya Family
Papaya

Parsley Family
Angelica, anise, black cumin, caraway seed, carrot, celery, chervil, coriander, cumin, dill, fennel, lovage, parsley, parsnip, star anise, sweet fennel

Passionflower Family
Passion fruit

Pepper Family
Black pepper

Pine Family
Juniper

Pineapple Family
Pineapple

Plum Family
Almond, apricot, cherry, nectarine, peach, plum

Pokeweed Family
Pokeweed
Pomegranate Family
Pomegranate
Poppy Family
Poppyseed
Protea Family
Macadamia nut
Purslane Family
Purslane
Rose Family
Black raspberry, blackberry, boysenberry, red raspberry, rose, strawberry, loganberry
Sac Fungi, (Class)
Maitake, morel, porcini, portobello, shiitake
Sea Vegetables Family
Agar, arrame, bladder weed, carrageen (Irish moss), dulse, laver, hijiki, kelp, kombu, nori, sea palm, wakame
Sesame Family
Sesame seed
Soapberry Family
Guarana, litchi, longan
Spurge Family
Tapioca
Sunflower Family
Artichoke, burdock, calendula, camomile, chicory, costmary, dandelion, endive, escarole, Jerusalem artichoke, lettuce, safflower, salsify, sunflower seed, tarragon
Tea Family
Tea
Truffle Family
Truffle
Walnut Family
Black walnut, butternut, English walnut, hickory nut, pecan
Water Chestnut Family
Water chestnut
Waterlily Family
Lotus

Yam Family
  Yam, Chinese potato
Yeast Family
  Yeast
Mollusk Class
  Clam, cockle, mussel, oyster, scallop
Shellfish Class
  Crab, crayfish, lobster, prawn, shrimp
Fish Class
  Barracuda, bluefish, bonito/tuna/mackerel,
  bullhead/catfish, carp, cod/haddock/pollack/whiting,
  eel, flounder/halibut, grouper/white bass/rock fish,
  herring, mullet, perch, pike, pompano, porgy/red
  snapper, salmon/trout/whitefish, sole, sturgeon,
  sunfish, swordfish
Amphibia Class
  Frog
Poultry Class
  Chicken, duck, egg, goose, pheasant, quail, turkey
Mammal Class
  Beef, cow's and goat's milk, lamb, pork, rabbit,
  venison, etc.

IDENTIFYING FOOD ALLERGIES

How can you find out if you might suffer from food allergies? The symptoms are wide ranging, but in general, if you have recurrent infections (such as ear, nose, or throat infections) or headaches (such as migraines or cluster headaches), you should suspect this problem. Other common symptoms include:

- fatigue
- anxiety, irritability, depression, or mental fogginess after eating
- asthma and shortness of breath
- skin rashes

- earaches
- swelling and joint pain
- frequent cystitis, vaginitis, or prostatitis
- digestive problems like bloating, gas, diarrhea, constipation
- frequent aches and pains
- itching after eating
- a constant sore throat
- dark circles under your eyes

Food allergies can be determined by a combination of methods. Prick or intradermal tests are one excellent indicator, and I find them extremely helpful in about 70 percent of my allergic patients. As previously explained, an extract of the offending food is scratched or injected under the skin to see if you develop a welt in response. The size of that welt is compared to a scratch test of a histamine or saline solution.

Total IgE blood tests measure your overall allergic state. As I mentioned earlier in this book, an IgE RAST test will measure the levels of IgE in your blood, and it can measure your responses to many common foods. This test gives a good indication of allergic potential, but it is not always accurate. It's most helpful in cases where there are a large number of suspected food allergies or where a potentially severe anaphylactic reaction to a scratch test is a possibility.

These tests give important information but still do not tell the whole story. They ought to be backed up with an elimination diet, in which suspected foods are eliminated and then reintroduced into the diet to see if symptoms occur.

TESTING FOR FOOD REACTIONS

If you have had symptoms or a food reaction in the past and wish to test them, you can systematically eliminate suspect foods from your diet and then reintroduce them, closely observing the results. You must be careful to monitor this process with your doctor, reintroducing the food in very tiny doses in the doctor's office. (I measure breathing capacity after these food challenges, using a peak flow meter.) Often the acute allergic response to a food after it has been eliminated is even stronger than the chronic response of day-to-day exposure. Do not attempt an unsupervised test of any food to which you might have an anaphylactic reaction.

A food diary can help you identify problem foods. Write down the foods you eat—all the foods you eat—as well as the symptoms you suffer each day. After a few days or a week, you may begin to see surprising patterns. For any elimination diet, it is wise to begin by eliminating the most common allergens (milk, wheat, soy, corn, peanuts). Any food that is eaten frequently may be a suspect. Try to eliminate junk foods first.

Although most patients can identify severe allergies, milder ones often go unnoticed. In addition, there may be foods that contain hidden allergenic substances. For example, tiramisu, a delicious dessert, contains almond extract and may cause problems for those sensitive to nuts.

After a week on an elimination diet, most food allergy sufferers feel better. They generally then add each suspected food back into the diet once every two to seven days (to allow for delayed reactions). In order to "challenge" your system with these foods, use them in their pure form. Use pure milk instead of ice cream, cream of wheat instead of bread, pure corn instead of corn tortillas, and so on.

Elimination diets need to be tailored to each individual.

For children, try to eliminate one food at a time, such as wheat or corn, and try to make appropriate substitutions. Use quinoa instead of wheat, for instance, since children can be so finicky.

I have several elimination diets that I recommend, if an elimination diet is needed.

Type I. This diet eliminates most common allergic foods. For one week, eliminate all:

- wheat
- corn
- yeast
- preservatives
- eggs
- chocolate
- sugar
- dairy products
- soy products
- coffee and tea

This may look far easier than it really is. Most prepared foods contain hidden traces of ingredients you cannot use. Wheat is not simply present in breads and cereals, it is used as filler in many soups, cold cuts and luncheon meats, and gravies. Corn is present in any product using corn oil or cornstarch—and that includes bacon, most candies, and sodas sweetened with "high fructose corn syrup." Eggs are used in pasta, milk is used in breads, yeast is used to make vitamins and is also present in everything from vinegars, pickles, and alcohol to malt products and moldy foods, including certain cheeses.

The easy way to approach this diet is to eat at home for a week, using only fresh foods: fresh fish and chicken, fresh vegetables, and carbohydrates such as rice and potatoes. This may require some advance planning in terms of shopping and cooking.

Type II. If you are feeling only slightly better after the first week or are still suffering from significant symptoms (wheezing, fatigue, digestive problems), eliminate the following foods. *Again, this need not be done all at once.* Try one food group at a time.

- bananas, berries, melons, apples, and all citrus fruits
- green peppers
- cabbage, brussels sprouts, and broccoli
- tomatoes
- all fish and shellfish
- all grains except rice
- all meats except lamb
- carrots
- eggplant
- all nuts
- herb teas

This is a very strict diet that allows you to eat lamb, sweet potatoes, melon, some vegetables (such as asparagus, green beans, green leafy vegetables), sea vegetables, rice, olive oil, and beets. You definitely won't starve, but you may be a bit bored. For variety, alternative grains such as spelt and amaranth can be tried (unless they are already a part of your diet, in which case you may have developed an allergy). Ninety-nine percent of those with food allergies will feel much better on this diet, and you can slowly reintroduce foods to your diet as you heal.

One patient of mine, a forty-two-year-old mother of three, said that everything she ate made her sick. We put her on a strict elimination diet and added back ten foods a month. It took three months before she was able to eat a varied diet again, but her health improved dramatically.

Type III. Very rarely, in extreme cases—those in which symptoms are severe and nothing seems to help—I will recommend an extremely regimented elimination diet. The patient will eat only rice for four days. Every four days a new food will be added, such as quinoa or pears. The foods least likely to cause allergies will be added first. This diet allows you to test about ten foods a month, but it is extremely tedious and recommended only in cases where the patient is in severe distress.

THE CANDIDA CONNECTION

You've probably heard or read about the theory that a proliferation of yeast can lead to uncomfortable symptoms, especially food allergies. Yeast sensitivity should be investigated in patients with numerous complaints, especially gas and bloating. I find overgrowth of yeast, or candida, to be a common cause of digestive problems and food allergies in my asthma patients. A stool test can be performed for yeast. A patient who scores high on this test usually does better when given an anti-yeast protocol. I have a patient who scored high but resisted yeast treatment. She went and had every other digestive test available and was given everything from antibiotics to Zantac, Flagyl, and bismuth. Nothing helped. Finally she began an anti-yeast protocol, and now says she hasn't felt so good in years.

Yet a stool test is not always a perfect indicator. Some of us are simply hypersensitive to yeast, even when the overgrowth is limited. I recently tested a woman with severe gas, bloating, and daily diarrhea whose yeast score on a stool test showed up as minimal. Yet, on a hunch, I put her on a trial course of nystatin, an antifungal antibiotic that is available only by prescription and is not absorbed outside the gastrointestinal tract. Her symptoms vanished within a week. She literally became a different person.

All of us have yeast in our bodies. It is when yeast overgrows, producing excess toxins and crowding out healthy bacteria, that we experience a problem. That overgrowth is common in a society where antibiotic use, which causes yeast to flourish, is practically a matter of rote. I know that as controversial as the so-called yeast syndrome may be in some quarters, yeast was a problem for me. I had taken many antibiotics for upper respiratory infections. When I began to treat myself for yeast, my digestive symptoms improved remarkably and immediately.

Yeast can grow in the gastrointestinal tract, the genital and urinary tracts, on the skin and nails, and in the mouth, nose, throat, and pharynx. If you are sensitive to yeast— either because you are allergic to yeast and molds or because you are sensitive to the toxins that yeast produces—you can suffer local and systemic reactions.

There are two main ways to fight yeast: one is through antifungal medications or herbs, and the other is through diet. Antifungal medications include nystatin, mentioned above, as well as some more serious prescription drugs that are absorbed throughout the body. These drugs belong to a class of antifungal medications known as azoles. Azoles are commonly used in over-the-counter yeast medications for women. For instance, there are the topical azoles clotrimazole (known as Gyne-Lotrimin) and miconazole (known as Monistat). Oral azoles are absorbed throughout the body and include ketoconazole (known as Nizoral), fluconazole (Diflucan), and itraconazole (Sporanox). Different azoles are effective for different strains of yeast and fungus, but they must be monitored carefully with blood tests because occasionally they can cause liver or kidney damage. Yet they can be quite useful in tough cases. One patient of mine, a thirty-five-year-old woman, says her life changed completely after I prescribed Sporanox. Other drugs did little for her, but the Sporanox was highly effective against whatever strain of yeast she was carrying.

For some reason, yeast-associated rashes are often misdiagnosed. A patient of mine had a persistent, disfiguring rash on her chin and cheeks after giving birth to her second child. (Pregnancy can sometimes exacerbate yeast, because high levels of progesterone in the body stimulate yeast growth.) A topical antifungal medication cleared it up in four days.

Nonprescription antifungals can also be very effective. I often recommend a combination of two powerful antifungal substances, artemesia annua and grapefruit seed extract. Artemesia annua, also known as wormwood, has been recently rediscovered because it is able to cure strains of malaria that have become resistant to the common prescription drugs. It also causes far fewer side effects. Artemesia annua happens to be an effective antifungal as well. Grapefruit seed extract is also a reliable, broadspectrum antifungal, and when the two are combined together, they work well to eliminate yeast in the digestive tract.

All antifungal medications, whether prescription or non-prescription, must be supplemented with beneficial bacteria such as acidophilus and bifido-bacteria, found in better brands of yogurt and also available commercially as supplements in health food stores. The supplements are best taken as refrigerated powders; a teaspoon is mixed in spring water and taken on an empty stomach in the morning, allowing the bacteria to colonize the entire digestive tract.

The Anti-Yeast Diet

An anti-yeast diet can bring relief from symptoms within a few weeks.

Foods and beverages to avoid include the following:

• All foods that contain sugar, yeast, or fermented products: honey, corn syrup, table syrup, cookies, candies, cakes, bread, crackers, muffins, cold cereals, canned fruit and juices, and fresh fruit—especially melons, bananas, and grapes

- All refined foods: pastas, breads, cakes, cookies
- Fermented foods or foods containing malt: soy sauce, vinegar, salad dressings, wines, champagne, certain cheeses, any products sweetened with malted barley
- Dried fruits
- Deli or processed meat
- All commercially prepared foods: pickled, smoked, or salted meats; sausages; salami; hot dogs; bacon; cured pork; aged cheeses; canned foods that contain citric acid

The following foods should be included in your anti-yeast diet:

- Vegetables: all
- Salads: all
- Fish: all
- Meats: beef, chicken, lamb, turkey, veal
- Whole grains: brown rice, corn, oats, amaranth, spelt, quinoa. (Note: If grains cause a reaction, eat them in small amounts. Some people need to temporarily cut down on all starch, including grains.)
- Vegetable and nut oils: olive, sesame, and peanut oil (if not allergic)
- Nuts and legumes: walnuts, cashews, garbanzo beans, string beans, peanuts. (Note: your diet should be tailored to your own individual needs. For instance, if you have an allergy to peanuts, no diet you eat should contain them.)
- Limited amounts of fruits and light cheese (farmer's and goat cheese), if tolerated well

TOXIC FOODS?

I never cease to be amazed at how many of my patients take an astonishing turn toward health when they eliminate allergenic foods from their diets. One of my patients repeatedly got bladder infections in the spring because she was allergic to pollens. She was actually experiencing cross-reactivity. We discovered that she could not tolerate certain fruits, but they created problems only in the spring. If she avoided those fruits during hay fever season, she had no recurrence of her cystitis.

I myself am extremely sensitive to certain foods, particularly to nuts and legumes. I know that if I eat one sesame seed by mistake, my mouth will swell, become inflamed, and itch. I can only imagine what that seed is doing to my gastrointestinal tract. (I can imagine that single tiny seed tracing a trail of red-hot inflammation all the way down my esophagus into my stomach and throughout my intestinal tract.) I find that for days after eating an allergenic food, I feel both flushed and fatigued whenever I eat anything at all, and I react more easily to other foods. (I suspect that the mucosa in my gut lining is temporarily inflamed and more porous.)

Sesame seeds and sesame oil are more commonly used now than in years past. Sesame oil is present in many salad dressings, in Mideastern foods like Halvah and humus, and even in some brands of margarine. That's why I am extremely careful about my diet. One mistake, and I suffer for it. You might be surprised how common mistakes are and how many foods contain hidden ingredients that can cause allergic reactions—or are just plain unhealthy for you.

Fake Foods: Or When Is a Cereal a Cookie?

Once you start paying attention to your food and what is in it, you will begin to realize how many foods are "fake." They are wearing a mask of "healthy" and "natural," but they are by no means healthy and natural. If you suffer from food allergies, you must be particularly careful of what substances foods may be hiding.

Did you know that your healthy can of tuna in spring water contains hydrolyzed plant protein—a flavor enhancer that is a derivative of soy? Anyone who is allergic to soy should be aware of this.

Your healthy cereal, which boasts of being all-natural, and containing no sugar, usually contains barley malt. Barley malt is a sweetener that has been fermented. It may be worse than sugar for those who are mold and yeast sensitive or who cannot tolerate fermented foods. You often find barley malt in "healthy" soy milk products as well.

Your favorite low-cholesterol food may be so high in fat that, although it contains not a gram of cholesterol, it raises your levels of cholesterol. Even ordinary table sugar, or sucrose, has been linked to increases in fat and cholesterol in a study in laboratory animals reported in an article in the journal *Nutrition* in the spring of 1994.

Your healthy snack of yogurt may be no better for you than pudding. Many commercial yogurts are loaded with sugar and, when tested, have low or absent levels of the beneficial bacteria, acidophilus and bifido-bacteria, that they claim to harbor.

Margarine, which was supposedly healthier than butter, actually raises levels of cholesterol and contains harmful trans-fatty acids and partially hydrogenated fats. These fats have been banned in Europe.

Vitamin-enriched breads and cereals can be of questionable benefit to those with allergies and sensitivities. I myself get nauseous every time I eat fortified cereals, whose flakes have been sprayed with vitamins. What are those vitamins made from? Some vitamins are manufactured from yeast, and yeast-sensitive individuals may be unable to tolerate them.

Popcorn, that healthy snack that you congratulate yourself on buying at the movie theater instead of candy bars, may be worse for you than a Milky Way. Seven out of ten moviegoers buy refreshments at the movies, often popcorn. It is usually popped in coconut oil, and a large popcorn contains an astounding eighty grams of fat; fifty of those grams are saturated fat. That's as much fat as six Big Macs from McDonald's. Some changes have been made since this information was first announced in the spring of 1994, but movie theater popcorn is still laden with fat.

Turkey breast is often not pure turkey, but an amalgam of fillers, fat, and turkey rolled into a loaf. Make sure you can actually see them cutting the slice of turkey off of a real bird.

Crabmeat that you purchase at the deli or salad bar is often imitation crab made of pollack, artificial coloring, artificial flavoring, and fillers. This concoction has caused several cases of food poisoning.

Plain M&M's are not plain. Like peanut M&M's, they also contain peanuts! For those who are allergic to peanuts—and some of us can die from a severe allergic reaction to peanuts—this can be literally life threatening.

Drugstore vitamins often contain much more than vitamins and minerals. A patient recently brought me her iron supplement, purchased in the neighborhood drugstore. It contained several different types of dyes, talcum powder, and fillers—along with iron!

HOW TO HEAL YOUR ASTHMA WITH FOOD

As I began to write this chapter, I realized what a great opportunity I had to reexamine my diet as I had done when I was so ill with asthma years ago. I have made many healthy changes in my eating patterns. Even so, today my practice is extremely busy, and it's easy for me to become a little too casual about my eating. I can dine in restaurants all too easily, especially when conducting business, and food in restaurants may not always be as pure as the waiter claims. I recently went out to lunch in a moderately expensive restaurant, ordered wild mushroom soup in chicken broth, and salad.

I asked the waiter, "What's in your soup? Is it fresh?"

"Yes, it's our own chicken stock."

That sounded delicious, but as I was raising the spoon to my lips, I saw the delivery man rolling a trolley through the kitchen piled high with giant, Andy Warhol–size cans of chicken stock. I recognized the brand. Some friends once served me homemade soup that, they assured me, contained nothing but pureed vegetables and chicken stock. I ate it and began to have an allergic reaction; it turned out they had used canned chicken stock—the same as the brand on the trolley—that contained hydrolyzed plant protein. This substance is made from soy and is a no-no for those who have a soy allergy.

Even a restaurant that is conscientious about its ingredients can pose a problem for the patient with food allergies. The cook may have prepared a meal with sesame oil, wiped the pan clean with a wet cloth, and may now be cooking your salmon steak on a pan still coated with sesame oil. If you're allergic to sesame, you may be in trouble.

On the other hand, home cooking may be safe, but it can be a complicated art—and I don't have a lot of spare time to master complicated recipes, or spend hours at the store combing the aisles for a pinch of this and a teaspoon of that. I wondered if, as a busy professional, would it be possible to prepare most of my own fresh, healthy, nonallergenic meals?

The answer is yes.

With a few simple purchases—such as a wok or some old-fashioned pots and pans, a breadmaker, a rice cooker or a pressure cooker, and a clay pot for baking succulent fish—cooking becomes not only a delight but quick and easy. Each day for the past week I've stopped at the fruit and vegetable stand or the supermarket after work. As I walk the aisles, I almost feel as if I'm grazing in a field of earthly delights. There's an almost primal sensation of pleasure as I choose whatever produce appeals to me that day: crisp broccoli, shiny red peppers, pale green snow peas, crunchy carrots, crinkly bunches of parsley or mint, aromatic garlic and onion, delicate baby asparagus, exotics like bok choy and special squashes. Fruits are just as beguiling and healthy: I rarely resist strawberries in season, and I enjoy the touch of sweetness seedless grapes and mandarin oranges add to vegetable dishes.

Healthy cooking is surprisingly easy. For instance, you can stuff a cornish hen with sage, rosemary, and garlic, wrap it in foil, and let it bake for forty minutes: a delicious ready-made meal.

Here's the latest news about the do's and don'ts of eating:

DO—eat fish. Studies have shown that fish oils are anti-inflammatory and appear to be helpful to asthmatics. (See chapter 7.)

DO—rotate your foods. Research shows that if you rotate your foods on a four-day schedule, you are less likely to suffer from food allergies.

DO—eat lots of garlic, onions, ginger, and cayenne. Garlic, onions, and ginger are antibiotic and boost the immune system. Cayenne is known to thin mucus and warm the body. These are good anti-asthma foods.

DO—eat lots of fruits and vegetables so that you get a hefty dose of healing phytochemicals every day.

DO—eat a lot of sea vegetables, which are high in protein and minerals. Arame is high in protein, potassium, iron, calcium, iodine, and vitamins A, B_1, and B_2. Dulse is high in iron, protein, calcium, phosphorus, iodine, potassium, magnesium, and vitamins A, C, B_6, B_{12}, and E. Hijiki is high in calcium (one portion supplies fourteen times the calcium in a glass of milk), along with phosphorus, iron, protein, and vitamins A, B_1, and B_2. Kombu is high in protein, iron, calcium, phosphorus, and vitamins A, B_1, B_2, and

C. Nori is high in protein, calcium, iron, potassium, magnesium, phosphorus, iodine, vitamins A, B$_2$, C, D, and niacin.

DO—eat whole grains and whole foods, which provide you with an assortment of nutrients, complex sugars, starches, and fiber.

DO—eat fruits and vegetables high in bioflavonoids, which have been shown to suppress histamine release. Some foods high in flavonoids include pineapple and citrus fruits.

DO—drink Oriental green tea, which contains small amounts of caffeine and methylated xanthines (known to dilate the bronchial tubes) as well as healing flavonoids. (Avoid teas if you are extremely mold-sensitive and react to residues of mold on tea leaves.)

DO—eat foods high in magnesium, such as tofu, wheat germ, swiss chard, spinach, amaranth, beets, broccoli, okra, bean sprouts.

DO—eat foods high in vitamin E, such as olive oil, soybeans, sunflowers, and wheat germ.

DO—eat foods high in special antioxidants such as vitamin C and beta-carotene, which have proven helpful in allergy and asthma. These include all fruits, dark leafy green vegetables like spinach and swiss chard, carrots, and squash.

DO—create healthy, natural spreads for whole grain breads. These can include overripe avocados, simply spread on whole grain toast; garlic butter created by infusing garlic in oil and freezing it; and nut butters made from raw, pure nuts.

DO—bake, broil, and steam food, or sauté it in a pan brushed lightly with a coating of oil.

DO—experiment with interesting grains such as millet, kasha (buckwheat), quinoa, amaranth, spelt, and kamut. Try hot cereals made of whole-grain brown rice, whole buckwheat, or whole oats. Eat whole-grain breads, sourdough breads, and sprouted grain breads. Try pastas made with Jerusalem artichoke, buckwheat, or brown rice.

DO—eat healthy condiments such as umeboshi plum (pickled plum that is good for digestion), gomasio (roasted sesame seeds and sea salt), lemon juice, fresh spices, pure Dijon mustard, low-sodium tamari (free of preservatives), and mirin (rice cooking wine).

DON'T—eat a diet heavy in trans-fatty acids and saturated fats. These fats are found in milk and milk products, animal meats, and in any food that contains artificially modified fats, including margarines, most commercial baked goods, commercial popcorn, and fried foods.

DON'T—eat foods that promote free-radical damage. That includes smoked and barbecued foods, foods grilled at high temperatures, and cured foods.

DON'T—eat denatured, refined foods such as simple sugars, white flours, cakes, cookies, white pastas, and any other so-called convenience foods.

DON'T—eat foods high in unsaturated vegetable oils such as corn and safflower oils. These contain high amounts of omega-6 fatty acids, which have been linked to inflammation. As some researchers have pointed out, the sharp increase in asthma in the last few decades may be due in part to the dramatic increase in our diet of harmful oils—oils known to be inflammatory.

Your Asthma Prevention Diet

Here is a general guideline for the healing foods to emphasize:

- Fish, especially fresh salmon, tuna, and mackerel
- Chicken or turkey (free range)
- All vegetables, particularly those rich in carotenes, such as green leafy vegetables, squash, and carrots
- Cruciferous vegetables, such as broccoli, cauliflower, cabbage, and brussels sprouts

- Apples, pears, and other fruits
- All fresh salads, salad greens, and sprouts
- Whole grains such as brown rice, millet, buckwheat, rolled oats, quinoa, amaranth
- Olive, canola, or flaxseed oil
- Nuts, sesame seeds, sunflower seeds
- Plain, low-fat yogurt with active acidophilus cultures
- All fresh spices, mint, ginger, cayenne
- Garlic and onions
- Occasional eggs

Remember not to eat any foods to which you are allergic.

What You Need to Start

A breadmaker allows you to determine exactly which ingredients are in your bread, and baking fresh bread this way takes very little time! You can be creative: add all kinds of flours, from buckwheat to rice to millet.

A wok, as far as I am concerned, is one of the best inventions for those of us who like creative (or even chaotic!) cooking. Anybody can be a cook with a wok. Yesterday I made a meal of broccoli, red peppers, snow peas, carrots, garlic, onions, asparagus, and bok choy. (I added three cloves of garlic to 2 tablespoons of olive oil and used vegetable stock to flavor this dish.) A side dish with a mixture of sweet, brown, and wild rice, along with pinto beans, made a completely healthy meal.

Ceramic or glass pots are my preference for cooking. Aluminum and iron can leach into food when used as cookware. For those of us who need extra iron, cast-iron pots can be fine, but at least 10 percent of the population tends to store excess iron. If you are already obtaining iron from foods and/or a supplement, you should know that excess iron has been linked to infections and lowered immunity.

Even stainless steel pots can pose a problem: a study found that any acidic food cooked in stainless steel leaches nickel from the pot, causing you to eat up to five times as much as the daily allowance of nickel. Since 10 percent of women are estimated to be sensitive to nickel, it may be wise to avoid stainless steel if you often cook with acidic foods such as tomatoes.

A clay pot is a handy purchase for those of you who love fish. Wrap the fish in special cooking paper, add spices and garlic, twist the paper, and bake it. When you take it out, it will be steaming hot and succulent.

Here are some cooking tips that I use almost daily:

1. Garlic is one of our healthiest foods. If you want garlic flavor but no garlic, cook it in oil and then remove the garlic pieces. Experiment with cutting the garlic (so that little pieces are in your food), lightly crushing it, or crushing it completely in a garlic press. Each method brings out a different flavor and intensity of garlic taste. Infuse garlic and herbs in olive oil overnight, and bake brown rice or whole grains with it for a delicious flavor.

2. You can also add ginger, onions, fennel root, or any other spices that you like to food. If you are cooking with chile peppers, begin with just a quarter of a tiny pepper and work your way up over time. Already you have a meal full of phytochemicals and antiinflammatory compounds, and you haven't even added the vegetables.

3. Begin with the foods that take longest to cook. Snow peas or peppers or broccoli, for instance, require more time than bok choy or parsley, which cook very quickly.

4. Experiment with fruits, which add beauty, color, and sweetness to a meal. Add seedless grapes, raisins, apples, pears, or mandarin oranges in the last minute of cooking.

5. Try different types of vinegar to flavor your meal—plum, rice, balsamic vinegar, or wine if you can tolerate it. The wine's alcohol will burn off in the heat, leaving only the flavor.

6. Make soups by steaming vegetables until they are soft-
ened, then making a puree in the food processor. Add soup
stock (chicken, fish, or vegetable). For creamy soups, add
low-fat yogurt. I love cauliflower and broccoli soup flavored
with garlic; squash soup with a dollop of low-fat yogurt and
a sprig of basil on top; or puree of carrot soup with ginger.

7. Try juicing vegetables and fruits as a snack, or to add
nutrition to a meal.

8. Look for new foods such as quinoa and amaranth.

Many individuals have a hard time shifting their diet at
first, especially if they feel dependent on or "addicted" to certain foods or sweets. After a few weeks, as you begin to develop a taste for and even a love of healthy eating, the changes
become easier. Patients who were terrified of giving up those
fat-larded cheeseburgers and french fries have come to me
months later waxing poetic about brown rice spiced with
natural herbs, garlic, and balsamic vinegar, and topped with
sautéed vegetables and melted mozzarella cheese. Working
parents may find this change especially difficult where their
children are concerned. But the effort is worth it.

A typical menu on any given day for me might include
oatmeal or organic eggs for breakfast, along with a slice of
whole-grain toast topped with organic apple sauce. Lunch
might be a colorful salad with varied greens and vegetables,
along with soup, chicken, or fish, a baked potato, and
cooked vegetables. Dinner might include anything from
cornish hens stuffed with sage and rosemary, to fish steamed
in a clay pot, as well as salads of greens and/or fruits, grains
ranging from rice to exotic types like quinoa and amaranth,
or soups made of steamed vegetables pureed in the food
processor and flavored with healthy, organic soup stocks.

Healthy soup stocks are available in your health food
store, or you can make them yourself and freeze them. Just
use chicken or fish, along with herbs and spices. Or go
vegetarian—throw vegetables in a pot: carrots, celery, pars-

ley, garlic, and onions. You may want to sauté the garlic and onions first in some olive oil to add flavor, or use arrowroot to thicken the broth.

HOW TO STAY HEALTHY ON THE ROAD

"Doctor Firshein, I've been following my healthy diet, and I feel much better," Bob, a computer programmer for a big company, told me. "I don't eat peanuts or corn, because I'm allergic to them. My wife and I have been cooking together, and I guess I must be a New Age man, because I'm enjoying it. But the problem is business lunches and dinners and travel. It's very hard to eat such a pure diet on the road! What can I do?"

I've heard that lament from many of my patients. Often they eat in restaurants, choosing what they think are healthy meals, and they feel ill afterward. I'm not surprised. There are estimated to be 2,000 commonly used additives in food, and many are not evaluated. Here are the main causes of adverse reactions in restaurants:

- Hidden ingredients. Some dishes contain substances to which you may be allergic.
- Sulfite, a preservative that comes in various forms and can cause problems for aspirin-sensitive asthmatics. Sulfites can cause bronchospasm, flushing, and itching, usually within fifteen minutes of eating the food. The problem is that a restaurant meal may contain as much as 200 milligrams of sulfite, while the average daily diet contains 2 to 3 milligrams. It can be hard for some of us to detoxify that high a level of sulfite.
- Monosodium glutamate, one of the most commonly known flavor enhancers, especially in Chinese restaurants. It began to be widely used in the 1960s, and the first documented case of "Chinese restaurant syndrome" occurred

in 1968. Certain people are unable to efficiently break down MSG and can react to it with symptoms ranging from burning pressure in the face, neck, and upper chest to bronchospasm.

- Tartrazine, a yellow dye to which asthmatics can be extremely sensitive.
- Tyramine, an ingredient in certain cheeses and red wine. It can cause a severe reaction, especially migraine headaches.

When eating out or on the road, I follow some guidelines that generally protect me. I try to eat only fresh, whole foods, such as fish, baked potatoes, and salad with lemon and olive oil on the side. Remember, restaurants may say their foods are free of additives, but this is not always so. Mashed potatoes may contain margarine or oils; soups may contain stocks with hidden additives and flavor enhancers.

A little ingenuity can go a long way. I was recently having a business lunch with a colleague who was in a big rush. He wanted to eat in the burger joint, and I had no choice but to go with him. I saw that the menu contained a Caesar salad with chicken, as well as a Greek salad. I asked the waiter for a combination without any salad dressing. The salad I was served was delicious—romaine lettuce, slices of baked chicken, calamata olives, olive oil, and balsamic vinegar on the side.

It's a good idea to find "safe" houses—restaurants that serve certain meals you know to be healthy and pure—in your hometown.

If you are traveling, bring a few reliable foods with you, such as tuna in spring water with no additives (available in health food stores), some whole-grain bread, fruits, vegetables, and nut butters. These basics can get you through plane travel and the first day in a new city. Ask your hotel if there is a refrigerator in your room.

Understanding the foods that can harm and help you can be one of the most important adventures of your life. We are, indeed, just beginning to understand the science behind Hippocrates' old maxim, "Let food be your medicine, medicine be your food."

And remember, when you are in a restaurant, don't be afraid to ask for what you want.

DOCTOR'S RECOMMENDATIONS FOR ACTION

1. Recognize that food can be medicine, and that more and more information is now available about plant chemicals that can help heal us. Eat foods that have known healing elements, such as soy, broccoli, cabbage, citrus fruits, garlic and onions, grapes, strawberries, parsley, and more.

2. Avoid foods that promote inflammation. These include fried foods, junk foods, smoked and barbecued foods, refined foods, foods high in unsaturated fatty acids (such as corn and safflower oils), or foods that contain partially hardened oils (such as margarine).

3. Try to eat a diet rich in fish, vegetables, fruits, salad greens, whole grains, olive and flaxseed oil, nuts, plain yogurt, fresh spices, and foods like garlic, ginger, onions, and cayenne.

4. Know the difference between anaphylactic (potentially fatal), allergic, and delayed allergic reactions. Be aware that some food allergies show up only at certain times—for instance, under stress, during menstruation, or during hay fever season.

5. Suspect food allergies if you suffer from common symptoms such as cyclical fatigue, moodiness, asthma, rashes, earaches, frequent infections, aches and pains, digestive problems, itching after eating, or dark circles under your eyes.

6. Ask your doctor for an overall IgE test to determine if you are in a highly allergic state.

7. Use a peak flow meter to test your response to foods. If your peak flow levels drop after eating a certain food, you may be allergic.

8. Identify your food allergies, either through laboratory testing and/or an elimination diet, and avoid any sensitizing foods. Suspect common allergens like wheat, soy, corn, and dairy products, as well as foods that you seem to crave and eat daily.

9. If you are allergic to a certain food, test yourself for allergies to other foods in the same family.

10. Ask your doctor to test you for candida (also known as fungus or yeast), which can irritate your intestinal lining and worsen food allergies. Work together with your doctor to eliminate candida through diet and antifungal medications or treatments.

11. Adopt a style of healthy cooking that utilizes healthy foods cooked simply. Make sure your kitchen contains the necessary essentials for healthy cooking: a wok, a breadmaker, a rice cooker or pressure cooker, and a clay pot for baking fish.

12. Be aware of restaurant meals and "healthy" supermarket foods. Try to eat fresh, whole foods in restaurants (fish, broiled meat, potatoes, rice, salads). Ask for all dressings on the side. Don't be afraid to ask how a food is cooked, and to request broiling or baking rather than frying.

13. For more information about food allergies and support, contact the Food Allergy Network, 4744 Holly Avenue, Fairfax, Virginia 22030.

CHAPTER NINE

Sick Air

Purifying the air you breathe is one of the most powerful and underestimated treatments for asthma. We inhale a pint of air fifteen times a minute. That's twenty-two thousand pints a day. Carried on those currents of air are all the chemicals, particles, and toxins of the modern industrialized world—forty-nine thousand chemicals, to be exact, along with nature's own pollens, grasses, and dust.

I believe the massive increase in both indoor and outdoor pollution is an important trigger for a simultaneous, dramatic rise in allergies and asthma around the world. Pollutants do more than damage the body. They actually sensitize the body to foreign particles of all kinds—from paint fumes to pollen. A century ago, Sir William Osler, a renowned physician, reported that asthma was a rare, mild condition in both children and adults, one that almost never resulted in death. Today, you regularly find asthmatics in emergency rooms gasping for their last breath.

In this chapter, you will learn about the major man-made toxins you can encounter indoors and outdoors. I'll explain the typical symptoms that different indoor toxins can cause, and how you can test for a wide range of unsuspected contaminants in your home and office. You'll find a detailed program for cleanup that will allow you, step by step, to create an environment that will begin to heal, not harm, your lungs.

Purifying your air can be as effective as taking certain medications. That is why I explain in detail all the toxins you can find in the air around you, and just how important it is to eliminate as many of them as you can. In my case, cleaning up the air in my home, above all, allowed me to return to New York City and live there quite comfortably in spite of the warnings of doctors who had treated me.

How do air pollutants worsen asthma? Consider ozone, a major health hazard that can cause coughing, painful breathing, and permanent lung damage. Right now ozone levels in at least ninety-six American cities are above the safety standard—and that's for individuals without asthma or other respiratory illness.

The fascinating link that is rarely mentioned is that ozone levels also worsen other allergies. One Canadian study published in *The Lancet* found that when asthma patients were challenged with "safe levels" of ozone, they became twice as sensitive to ragweed and grass. The ozone concentration was .12 parts per million per hour, the level approved by the Environmental Protection Agency (EPA). Apparently ozone worsens allergies by increasing production of inflammatory chemicals in the body. In one British study at St. Bartholomew's Hospital in London, patients were exposed to ozone in sealed chambers for four hours and then exposed to pollens. They had a threefold increase in sneezing and mucus production in reaction to pollen, and a fivefold increase in inflammatory chemicals in their bloodstreams.

The sad fact is that our air is sick, and it is making us sick. The Clean Air Act of 1990 introduced regulations that would remove 56 billion pounds of pollutants from the air each year. That number is so immense it's nearly unimaginable. The question is, how many hundreds of billions of pounds of pollutants will still be left? The Global Environment Monitoring System (GEMS) estimates that 1.2 billion city dwellers are now being exposed to air pollution so toxic it actually damages their health permanently. Up to sixty thousand Americans are killed each year by soot, according to a recent study by the EPA. Yet the dangers of soot were totally ignored until this study caused a flurry of media attention in 1993.

Who do you think is most at risk? Children and the elderly who are already suffering from respiratory disease, and asthmatics of all ages are the most susceptible. The raw data speaks for itself: asthma statistics have jumped from 6.8 million Americans in 1980 to 12.4 million today, and death rates have nearly doubled. Certain cities are even worse: the mortality rate is double the national average in Chicago, and triple in New York. Worldwide statistics are about the same.

Deaths from air pollution rival deaths caused by some types of cancer. A recent study conducted by the Harvard School of Public Health and published in the *New England Journal of Medicine* tracked over eight thousand residents in six different states for sixteen years. The result? They found a strong relationship between pollution and death rates—especially with deaths from respiratory problems and heart disease. There was a direct link between deaths and the pollution generated by diesel trucks and buses, factory smokestacks, boilers, and wood-burning fireplaces. In fact, mortality rates could be predicted merely by looking at levels of air pollution in cities.

The enemy in our air is invisible. The most lethal particles are microscopic "suspended particulates," commonly known as soot. These toxins are so minuscule they can easily penetrate deep into the lung and evade the immune system, causing lasting tissue damage. Once soot is inhaled, it is difficult for the body to remove because it is so small and so deeply embedded. A typical particle of soot is less than 10 microns in diameter. Compare that to a human hair, which is 70 microns wide.

City dwellers are not the only victims of sick air. Today's pollution knows no boundaries. By-products of industry have been found at the north and south poles. Even the Grand Canyon, a natural wonder set far from America's cities, is periodically obscured by polluted air blown over from neighboring states, limiting visibility for disappointed visitors and honeymooners. Even weather can contribute. In June of 1994, a severe thunderstorm in London caused emergency room visits to increase by ten times. Similar episodes have occurred in Australia. Thunderstorms may cause pollens and pollutants to spread.

Air pollution not only damages health, it is expensive. A 1989 study by the EPA estimated that in the city of Los Angeles alone, $9.4 billion would be saved each year in health costs if the city merely met the federal government's clean air standards, and $14.3 billion would be saved a year if the city met California's somewhat stricter standards. How much could be saved nationally if every major city cleaned up its air?

Perhaps you are thinking that if the air outside is so bad, you ought to retreat indoors to a safe place. Unfortunately, indoor air pollution can be up to ten times worse than outdoor pollution, occasionally reaching levels that would be illegal outdoors. A 1996 study of inner-city children in New York found they had double the risk of asthma, not simply because of air pollution, but because of indoor pollution from cockroaches, smoke, and poor ventilation. The EPA has listed indoor pollution as one of the top environmental threats Americans face today. Radon (a deadly radioactive gas often emitted into homes from polluted ground sources) alone is believed to cause up to twenty thousand lung cancer deaths a year. Aside from radon, consider the typical American house: caulked and insulated, filled with particleboard, paints, and synthetic carpets that emit toxic formaldehyde fumes, decorated with floor tiles containing asbestos, conditioned with humidifiers that are breeding bacteria, doused daily with a whole panoply of cleaning chemicals.

The typical office or hotel is no better. I recently went to a convention in Boston where my hotel room had just been cleaned—in other words, sprayed and scrubbed with chemical solvents. The moment I walked in I was assailed with chemical odors and began to wheeze. The hotel was kind enough to air out my room and bring in an air purifier. Nonetheless, my airways were constricted the entire weekend.

Remember Legionnaires' disease—the deadly outbreak of illness at a hotel in Philadelphia in the midseventies? It was caused by bacteria carried in air-conditioning systems. Our buildings have not improved much since that disaster. Today, the World Health Organization estimates that at least 30 percent of all buildings circulate polluted air.

Problems in tightly sealed office buildings have become so pervasive that such buildings have been dubbed "sick" themselves. Sick building syndrome, as it is called, first came to national attention when thirty employees at the EPA became chemically sensitive and suffered health problems after new carpeting was installed. New carpets typically contain more than twenty different chemicals designed to kill microbes, resist stains, and hold colors. That ironic and tragic occurrence eventually spurred the EPA to lobby Congress to officially recognize an illness known as "multiple chemical sensitivity."

Not only are some buildings sick, some airplanes can be as well. Air is recirculated, chemicals are released from synthetic materials, and bacterial infections can be passed. An April 1996 study in the *New England Journal of Medicine* found that one stewardess and several passengers became infected with tuberculosis while on a flight, because of the coughing of one infected passenger in the rear.

If asthmatics are the proverbial canaries in the coal mine—the first to react to toxic air—they suffer for it in more ways than one. Asthmatics often feel as if they are living in a world of "hot spots," places they just cannot go without feeling sick. They may suffer in a home where air is circulating poorly, become sick on a city street when exposed to a cloud of diesel fumes, or have difficulty working in high-rise buildings whose windows cannot be opened. It may seem that few places are safe.

Yet as bad as the quality of our air may be, there is much that can be done to improve it. In my own case, changing the air I breathed at home and the office was one of the most important and difficult steps I took toward health. Once I was breathing purer air on a regular basis, I was able to withstand many other assaults in my environment.

It's amazing to me how often patients' problems clear up when they change their environment—and how varied the different contaminants can be. For Veronica, a thirty-two-year-old mother, the culprit was dust. She came to me because her two sons, four and seven years old, suffered from severe allergies and asthma. Her home turned out to be a haven for dust, to which both of her sons were severely allergic. Her family's living space was carpeted throughout; her younger son's room was filled with stuffed animals; wool blankets were used on the bed, along with feather-filled pillows. My cleanup prescription for Veronica: roll up the carpets, put mattress covers on the bed, use foam pillows and washable cotton blankets, get rid of the stuffed animals, and buy air purifiers for both sons' rooms. Within six weeks, the boys were sleeping through the night and breathing much easier. Their runny noses and coughs disappeared, and they were able to begin steadily reducing their asthma medication.

Another patient of mine, Tad, a forty-two-year-old financial analyst, was struck ill by something entirely different: hypersensitivity to molds. He had just built a new home in a beautiful, wooded area of eastern Long Island, but he did not waterproof it. That year he began to get so sick with asthma that he was constantly using cortisone sprays and bronchodilators. He was using up to 25 puffs of cortisone a day, which is more than three times the recommended dose. He had fallen ill with several cases of bronchitis and severe asthma attacks over a two-year period, was prescribed large doses of antibiotics, and felt dragged out and tired for weeks afterward. When he came to me, he was both depressed and frantic, and at one point, his physician placed him on anti-depressants.

"I'm not able to concentrate like I used to," he told me. "I can't stop wheezing. I don't sleep well at night."

As soon as I evaluated his home as part of a housecall I made, I could immediately identify the distinct odor of mold. I placed mold plates—devices that identify different molds in the environment—throughout the house, and the mold counts that came back from the laboratory read: "Too numerous to count."

Tad found it hard to believe his new home was making him sick, but an inspection confirmed my suspicions. Water from the soil was seeping directly into the walls. We later learned his foundation had been placed without the use of any sealant, which would normally prevent water seepage. He now has temporarily built ditches around his home to collect water, while waiting for his home to be properly sealed. Not surprisingly, the mold counts in his home have dropped and his symptoms have dramatically improved. He is already down to eight puffs a day.

A third patient, Susan, had frequent asthma attacks, accompanied mysteriously by chills. It turned out that her corner office had recently been remodeled after a promotion, and new carpeting had been laid down. When I did an evaluation, I found that so much glue had been applied to the bottom of the carpeting that it was actually seeping through the fabric, and one could see a dark border of stains around the edge. Under the carpet, the glue was still moist and sticky, though it had been laid down weeks ago. Ventilation in Susan's office was poor, so she spent her days breathing in toxic fumes. Once we understood the problem, she transferred to another office while hers was stripped of carpeting and cleaned. Her asthma attacks disappeared.

As you will see when you read on, deciphering the contaminants in the air you breathe is like solving a mystery. The clues are often completely hidden to the average asthma sufferer. Solving the mystery can also be an adventure, with surprising benefits.

PART 1:
INDOOR AIR: ARE YOUR HOME AND OFFICE SICK?

Five years ago, Maria, a thirty-eight-year-old patient of mine, and her husband, Vadim, remodeled the interior of their New York brownstone. They used common building materials, including forty-three sheets of particleboard, which is made of wood chips held together by glues and resins that can emit formaldehyde gas. Within a few weeks, Maria became sick with what she later described as a "weird flu." She developed a sinus infection that wouldn't go away, burning eyes, a cough, and a tight chest, along with aching muscles. As the days passed, she got worse, not better. Her husband finished the remodeling, including their new upstairs bedroom, and Maria found herself coming home from work each day feeling tired, collapsing into bed, sleeping the sleep of the dead for twelve or thirteen hours—and waking feeling even worse.

When Maria came to me, I suspected formaldehyde poisoning, since I knew that fresh particleboard could emit toxic amounts of the gas. The health department tested her home and confirmed their fears, and so Maria and Vadim were forced to hire a contractor to rip out the entire forty-three sheets. Maria lived with her sister during that time and began a treatment program to strengthen her immune system. She moved back into her home and is doing well today, except that she is still sensitive to formaldehyde and cannot spend more than a few minutes in new buildings or newly carpeted homes without having an attack of wheezing, sneezing, burning eyes, and fatigue.

Your home or office can be a source of countless contaminants—from man-made chemicals to bacteria, molds, and dust. In most homes, toxins are built in, and modern building materials will typically emit fumes from about thirty to forty compounds into the air for years. The technical term for this is outgassing. According to Dr. William J. Rea (a surgeon who operated on John Connally after he was injured during the Kennedy assassination), these synthetic environmental toxins are affecting a good 20 percent of the population. Rea claims that indoor air pollution is the worst source of pollution in our environment. Dr. Rea runs one of the biggest treatment programs in the country, headquartered in Dallas, for victims of environmental illness.

At present, there are no guidelines for air safety in homes and very few guidelines for offices, particularly where chemical contaminants are concerned. Several different agencies—the EPA, the National Institute of Occupational Safety and Health (NIOSH), and the Occupational Safety and Health Administration (OSHA)—have all established separate guidelines for schools, businesses, and industries. Yet exposure levels called safe by these agencies are quite capable of causing health problems, especially for asthmatics. I've seen it happen again and again in my practice.

The National Academy of Science has stated that levels of contaminants in homes should be far lower than in the workplace. After all, most of us spend at least twice as much time in our homes as we do in the office. According to government studies, fresh air is supposed to circulate in a building at least 2.5 times an hour, but most ventilation systems in homes and offices allow about a 10 percent exchange of air over any given hour.

There are so many airborne contaminants in a typical home or office that to describe them all would be a book in itself. Most of these toxins cause free-radical damage, which harm your body's cells and immune system and trigger mutations in genes. A so-called "healthy" home now contains trichloroethane, xylene, ozone, bacteria, fungus, mold, toluene, glass fibers, dust, petrochemicals, lead, benzopyrene, radon gas, asbestos, sulfur dioxide, nitrogen oxide, hydrogen cyanide, carbon monoxide, plastics, chemical dyes, pesticides, benzene, styrene, phenol, formaldehyde, hydrocarbons, solvents, urethane, vinyl flooring, paints, finishes, glues, resins, caulks, wood preservatives, and more. Some of these contaminants are more harmful than others.

What follows are the most common airborne contaminants that you are likely to find in your home and office, along with the typical symptoms they cause. I have divided them into two classes: chemical and natural. Chemicals might include contaminants like formaldehyde and carbon monoxide. Natural contaminants include living things like molds and bacteria.

Common Chemicals in the Home

Formaldehyde. This is one of the most deadly gases around, and it's everywhere. Six billion pounds are manufactured in this country each year, to be used in fabrics, oil-based paints, paper towels, detergents, grocery bags, soft plastics like shower curtains, toiletries, cosmetics, and countless other products. Formaldehyde is known to bind with certain immune-system cells, creating a chemical antigen that can cause allergic-type reactions. Although formaldehyde has been declared by the EPA to be a probable cause of cancer in humans, products containing formaldehyde make up an astounding 8 percent of the U.S. gross national product. That's because it's easy and inexpensive to manufacture, and it's also incredibly effective as a binder and preservative.

Formaldehyde is used in almost all perfumed soaps, including bubble bath (which may be why some of my asthmatic patients complain that they don't feel well after "luxuriating" for a half-hour in a steamy bubble bath). It's a prime constituent of particleboard, which has been used to construct the homes of over 50 million Americans. According to studies conducted at Ball State University in Indiana, even five years after particleboard has been installed, it can release formaldehyde levels of .3 parts per million into the air. At a mere third of that—.1 part per million—humans will suffer from sore throats, headaches, fatigue, sinus problems, eye irritation, chest pains, difficulty breathing, and other symptoms. Safe levels are generally considered to be at .03 and below, but each state has established different safety levels and they vary widely.

It's difficult to determine just what safe levels of formaldehyde might be. NIOSH guidelines are .1 part per million parts of air; the federal government recommends .4 parts per million, and the Department of Housing and Urban Development (HUD) says that housing materials can safely emit .3 parts per million. I'm concerned that guidelines about a poisonous gas are so erratic. Formaldehyde poisoning is known to cause an enormous range of debilitating symptoms, from headaches to fatigue, central nervous system damage, wide-ranging allergies, asthma, and sinus problems.

To detect formaldehyde in the home, I use a device called DynoMeter (see resource section on p. 237 for supplies and services mentioned in this chapter). It is a portable syringe. You draw in air around potential hot spots—from carpet to particleboard to fabric-covered furniture and drapery—and the device will tell you how many parts per million of formaldehyde it has registered. Another tester that is widely available is the 3M 3720 Formaldehyde Monitor, which costs about forty dollars and is hung in the house for a few hours before being returned to the laboratory.

Sometimes I am truly surprised by what I find. One patient of mine suffered from nocturnal asthma. I tested her bedroom and found nothing. Then I noticed she was using an electric blanket. We turned it on, and as it was heating up, dangerous formaldehyde levels were emitted. Her blanket was emitting four times the recommended safety levels. The gas leaked from the plastic heating coils, and my unsuspecting patient would pull the blanket over her face on cold winter nights and receive a "direct hit" of formaldehyde all night long!

To correct the problem, sources of formaldehyde often need to be removed. That can entail time and heartache if it means ridding your home of new carpet or fabric-covered furniture, but the dramatic improvement in your health and lungs will be worth it.

Before actually removing carpet that is outgassing formaldehyde and other chemicals, you can try a stopgap measure: Rent a commercial steam-cleaner (not a rug shampooer) and a steam-cleaning concentrate without deodorant. Steam clean the carpet twice. Then use a carpet sealer such as Carpet Guard. The fumes may be far less potent.

In addition, try to avoid building with formaldehyde products in the future. In particular, avoid medium-density fiberboard (MDF), which is about three times as potent as particleboard. MDF is often used as a core material under plywood or veneers in furniture. Use solid wood whenever possible.

TWO NOVEL WAYS TO CLEAN SICK AIR

Indoor air that is toxic because of formaldehyde or any other volatile chemical can sometimes be treated with innovative techniques. One is an ozone machine, which is available through mail-order catalogues such as Allergy Control Products. The price can vary, but generally ozone generators cost several hundred dollars. Although breathing in ozone (as you will read in a moment) can be harmful to the lungs, the specialized use of ozone-generating machines can actually clean up sick air. They are best used when you are out of the room. Ozone is a highly reactive molecule that will bind with other airborne chemicals and neutralize them, turning them to carbon dioxide or water. It is important to ask a specialist to assist with this method, and be sure not to stay in the room while the ozone machine is running.

Another method that can work for soft plastics that emit toxins is to "bake" a room. This involves heating up the room (through portable heaters if necessary) to 90 degrees or higher. Just as heat hardens ceramics, it can dry out soft plastics so they will not outgas. (By the way, this method can be used outdoors for products like shower curtains and other plastic products. Open the product and leave it out in the sun for the day.) Again, this treatment method must be undertaken by a specialist, so that no damage occurs to the products or home.

Radon. Radon is a colorless, odorless, radioactive gas that is naturally found in soil at low levels. Radon becomes a problem when it becomes trapped in buildings and builds up to dangerous levels. In the presence of pollutants, the charged molecules of the gas attach themselves to dust, soot, or smoke, and then you breathe them deeply into your lungs. The particles continuously emit radiation, which damages the lungs by causing the production of free radicals (discussed in chapter 2), further complicating asthma.

The EPA guideline is 4 picoCuries of radon per liter of air. Levels often increase during summer, when soil becomes dry and porous, releasing more gas. Radon is especially damaging to lungs and has been linked to lung cancer, along with leukemia and other cancers. Countless homes have been found to harbor dangerous levels of radon. A radon detecting kit with an alarm and activated charcoal is manufactured by Alpha Energy Laboratories. The kit is exposed to in-home air for two to seven days. If the lab detects high levels, more sophisticated testing should follow.

In order to clean a home of radon, cracks in floors, walls, and foundations must all be sealed, along with all ground piping. The EPA lists over a thousand contractors who specialize in radon testing and cleanup. I recommend radon testing for all homes.

Carbon monoxide. A colorless, odorless gas that is the by-product of kerosene, gas heaters, leaking chimneys and furnaces, wood stoves and fireplaces, gas appliances, and auto exhaust. Carbon monoxide interferes with oxygen delivery in the body, and since asthmatics are chronically oxygen deprived, it can have disastrous effects on their health. Low levels of carbon monoxide can cause fatigue and heart problems; higher levels can exacerbate asthma and cause headaches, weakness, confusion, and nausea. People who suffer from carbon monoxide poisoning often mistake their symptoms for the flu. Special kits are available to test for carbon monoxide, and devices can be installed in the kitchen or near a gas heater so that an alarm will sound if carbon monoxide levels become dangerous. I like to test for low levels of carbon monoxide as well.

You can minimize carbon monoxide in your home by monitoring all gas appliances, using gas space heaters and furnaces that are vented to the outdoors, keeping fireplace flues open, and hiring a professional to annually inspect and maintain central heating systems that are gas based. Check your garage as well. Many homes and some offices are connected to their garages, and car owners will warm up their cars in winter months for fifteen or twenty minutes, while the tailpipe spews carbon monoxide exhaust into the air.

This happened at a major university hospital, where many employees and patients were falling ill with respiratory problems, fatigue, and flulike symptoms. Some of the ventilation system's intake valves, which brought fresh air into the hospital, were actually located in the hospital garage. Employees were being poisoned by carbon monoxide, probably because of an architect who didn't know better.

Nitrogen dioxide and carbon dioxide. Nitrogen dioxide is released when fuel is burned—most commonly in kerosene heaters, gas stoves and furnaces, and boilers. The gas can cause eye, nose, and throat irritation and impaired lung function, and it can also trigger respiratory infections. Even a small amount of the gas can cause increased mucus production, shortness of breath, cough, and headaches. Studies have shown that nitrogen dioxide can depress the immune system (specifically the macrophages, which are like the Pac-Men of the immune system, gobbling up invaders). Cleanup is the same as for carbon monoxide.

Carbon dioxide levels can be too high in homes or offices that are not properly ventilated. High carbon dioxide levels put greater stress on an asthmatic's lungs, which are already partially starved for oxygen. Other symptoms can include headaches, dizziness, increased heart rate, and high blood pressure. Improved ventilation is a necessity, especially installing a source of fresh air intake.

Simple devices are available to detect for both these airborne gases.

Ozone. The health effects of ozone depend on where it is in the environment. In the upper reaches of our atmosphere, it provides a protective layer that filters out ultraviolet radi-

ation. In our immediate air, however, ozone is usually a
health hazard (an exception are ozone-generating machines,
discussed on page 203). This colorless gas is a major component of smog. Produced by photocopy machines, laser
printers, and countless other electrical products that are
common in the office and home, low levels of ozone can produce coughing, while moderate levels can trigger chest
pain, nasal congestion, and shortness of breath. However,
asthmatics are known to be highly sensitive to ozone, and
the gas may worsen bronchitis and emphysema as well.
More ozone forms at high temperatures, so the hotter the
day, the greater the buildup of ozone.

Solutions include opening the windows to make sure
fresh air ventilates the room and making sure ozone-
generating machines are not placed in small, windowless
rooms.

Pesticides. In the early 1940s, the first modern pesticide
was developed by Germany as a nerve gas for use in World
War II. Now over a hundred thousand chemical compounds
have been developed for use as pesticides. Considered to be
major indoor and outdoor health hazards by many public
health officials, many of the products have been banned.
These synthetic compounds kill everything from insects to
rodents and fungi. They are sold as sprays, crystals, sticks,
powders, foggers, bombs, liquids, and balls.

Pesticide vapors can cause eye, nose, throat, and lung irritation, along with immune system and central nervous system damage.

Avoid pesticides whenever possible. If exposed indoors,
ventilate the area immediately. If you garden, try to control
pests with natural methods, which include planting diverse
species, making sure healthy soil is available to foster hardy,
pest-resistant plants, and using "natural" pesticides that are
less harmful than some of the common, widely used commercial sprays. Make sure to wash thoroughly after working
near pesticides, and try to protect yourself with clothing,

gloves, glasses, and breathing masks if you actually are required to spray the chemicals yourself.

Lead. Though lead was banned from paint in 1978, lead dust is still a problem in many homes and offices, especially when owners decide to renovate. When lead paints get old, they tend to buckle and flake. Lead poisoning can cause permanent damage to the brain and to the nervous, circulatory, digestive, and respiratory systems. Lead dust is a natural by-product of lead paint oxidizing and chalking. Over the years, the paint tends to flake, creating a chalky dust that is extremely fine and settles quickly. An asthmatic can be particularly vulnerable to lead dust settling in sensitive, already inflamed lungs.

Lead paint should never be sanded or burned off. During renovation of lead-painted walls or ceilings, professionals familiar with the hazards should be called in, and homeowners should temporarily live elsewhere. Workers need to be protected with respirators, glasses, and special clothing. After renovation, a high-efficiency particle air (HEPA) vacuum needs to be used to thoroughly remove any remaining dust.

You can test your home for air contamination (see the resource section at the end of the chapter).

Mercury. Mercury poisoning can result in chest pain, difficulty breathing, fever, headaches, and central nervous system damage. On August 20, 1990, the EPA banned the use of mercury in interior paints because of poisoning from inhalation. Houses painted before 1990, especially when undergoing renovation, can release significant amounts of mercury dust. (By the way, there is still a fiery controversy over mercury amalgams used in fillings in teeth. Some dentists and health professionals maintain that these fillings can release significant amounts of mercury vapor during chewing.)

For information on testing for mercury vapor in the home, see RCI in *Resources*.

Chlorine. Many of my patients complain about problems

while taking a shower, and I find two culprits. Molds and chlorine. Chlorine is a widely used disinfectant, and when it was first added to water around 1900, water-borne diseases were virtually eliminated. However, chlorine is known to interact with other chemicals to produce by-products that can damage the immune system. Some of the highly toxic chlorine compounds you may find in your drinking water include, among others, chloroform, chlorodibromomethane, trichloroethylene, tetrachloroethylene, chlorophenols, chlorobenzenes.

During a hot shower, the body absorbs chlorine through the open pores of the skin and by breathing in chlorine-laced steam. For an allergic asthmatic, someone who is sensitive to various toxic compounds, chlorine inhalation can be a problem. I recommend buying filters for the shower and tap to purify all water sources.

Volatile organic chemicals. If I had more time, I would discuss every volatile organic chemical individually—chemicals like ammonia, acetic acid, benzene, acetone, ethanol, methanol, and others that are remarkably common in cleaners, shampoos, disinfectants, solvents, sealants, aerosol sprays, air fresheners, paint thinners and removers, and countless other products. Gases and vapors from these chemicals can cause throat and lung irritation, along with burning of the eyes and nose, nausea, dizziness, chest pain, and headaches. Long-term exposure can sensitize the lungs to other toxins and is suspected to be a cause of cancer.

Paint can be a source of volatile chemicals. Oil-based paints contain thirty to forty volatile chemicals. Water-based paints contain far less—from twelve to fifteen—but they still contain biocides, which prevent mold from growing and can cause asthma in sensitive individuals. Some custom paints are made without biocides. You can also use natural paints from Europe or old-fashioned milk paint—or even plaster walls with no finish at all.

One patient of mine, Veronique, a twenty-eight-year-old painter who had moved to New York from Paris, began to suffer wheezing, fatigue, and burning of her eyes. She had already been diagnosed as asthmatic when she came to see me.

I asked her about ventilation in her studio, to which she replied cheerfully, "Oh, yes, sure, it is ventilated." When I suggested an evaluation, I found one tiny fan in the corner. The fumes from benzene, paint thinner, and oil-based paints were so intense I had trouble staying in the room. I explained to her that she was breathing in the toxic outgassing of many organic solvents.

Because she could not move, our solution was to build a HEPA air filter with two arms, modeled after those used for chemistry desks. One funnel went over her paint set and another over the painting. A better ventilator was installed in the window, and a general HEPA filter was used for the room itself. Within a few weeks, her symptoms had abated dramatically.

Asbestos. The word *asbestos* actually means inextinguishable, and asbestos is a name for a group of indestructible mineral fibers. A strand of hair is twelve hundred times wider than an asbestos fiber, which is so light and narrow it can elude the natural defenses of the body. Asbestos fibers are known to pierce cells in the lung, and although the body's immune system tries to eat them up and dispose of them, it cannot. Asbestos, in short, permanently damages the lungs. One form of asbestos poisoning, mesothelioma (cancer of the lining of the lungs) has been known to kill children within three years of their falling ill. Usually, however, asbestos is a silent killer that shows up ten to forty years after exposure. In the case of asthmatics, whose airways are already inflamed and damaged, asbestos only adds fuel to the fire.

Houses built before 1970 may contain potential danger areas of asbestos. Asbestos is present in fire-retardant sheeting, cement asbestos board, vinyl products, insulation of all sorts (for furnaces, pipes, interior ducts, and more), and in fireproofing materials. You may find it in the insulation of many steam and hot-water pipes, around furnace ducts, as thermal insulation around floors and walls, in vinyl adhesive, older lamp sockets, and old-fashioned "knob and tube" wiring and fuse boxes. Even in-home appliances such as portable dishwashers, toasters, slow cookers, clothes dryers, broilers, and popcorn poppers contain asbestos. Most of these sources are not hazardous unless the asbestos is disturbed or friable.

In 1986, the EPA banned the production of most asbestos products. Nonetheless, if you suspect that your home contains a lot of asbestos products, you can sample the air with a simple air cassette and air pump. Asbestos around a pipe may look like a chalky, hard covering. If you notice that it is flaking, do not touch it. Call in a professional. Air samples are collected and sent to a laboratory for analysis. Asbestos hazards can be minimized by encapsulating dangerous sources (applying a liquid material that then hardens to seal against the release of fibers). I recommend hiring a professional to seal asbestos rather than removing it. Removal of asbestos needs to be carried out by professionals using respirator masks and safety clothing, and as in the case of lead, homeowners need to stay away during the cleanup. Afterward, a HEPA vacuum needs to be used and a followup air sample taken.

The Consumer Product Safety Commission offers a hotline for information about asbestos removal. Call 800-638-2772, ext. 300.

Common Natural Contaminants in the Home and Office

Molds and bacteria. A large percentage of my asthma patients are sensitive to molds, and unfortunately even the briefest exposure can set off an attack. Perhaps the most common response to airborne molds is respiratory irritation. Symptoms range from watery eyes to sinus congestion, irritation of the respiratory system, and acute asthma attacks. Occasionally mold spores can cause a form of pneumonia known as pneumonitis. It is actually a hypersensitivity reaction to molds, and symptoms include tightness in the chest, fever, chills, fatigue, and coughing.

Bacteria, such as the one that caused Legionnaires' disease, can cause severe respiratory illness and even death. Bacteria are generally not responsible for allergic problems, whereas molds often cause a hypersensitivity response that is related to allergies and tends to be chronic. For that reason, I focus mainly on molds when considering microbes in the home and office.

Molds that grow in homes and offices often send out spores that may land on the skin and are also breathed in through the nose and mouth. Mold spores irritate the human body, but most of the molds do not actually grow inside us. (An important exception is candida albicans, a common cause of yeast infections. A few other molds, such as coccidioides, can cause infections as well, but they are far rarer.)

COMMON MOLDS

Here is a list of the most common molds and their favorite breeding places:

Alternaria tenuis: Grows on plants and is one of the most common causes of allergy.

Aspergillus fumigatus: Grows in the soil, on damp hay, grain, fruit, and sausage. It's the most common cause of respiratory disease in humans.

Basidiomycetes: Grows on grains but is most commonly found outdoors.

Candida albicans: An airborne yeast that is found not only in the soil but in the human body—most commonly in the throat, respiratory tract, digestive tract, and genitals.

Chaetomium: Grows on soil, damp paper, fabric, and straw.

Cladysporium: Grows on plants, leather, and wood. A common cause of respiratory problems.

Curvularia: Grows on tropical soils, tropical crops, and some birds. It is easily airborne.

Epicoccum: Grows on soil, plants, uncooked fruit, paper products, and human skin. Commonly causes runny nose and congestion.

Geotrichum and gliocladium: Similar molds that grow on soil, damp canvas, wood, and paper products.

Helminthosporium: Grows on cereal grains, including corn, rye, wheat, and oats.

Hormodendrum: Grows on leather, rubber, cloth, wood, paper, and decomposing plants. A common cause of respiratory problems.

Mucor: Grows in the soil and around barns and barnyards.

Penicillium notatum: Grows on fruits, breads, cheeses, and other foods.

Phoma: Grows on paper, magazines, books, and some paints and plants.

Pullularia pullulans: Grows on plants and decaying plants.

Rhizopus: Grows on bread, cured meats, root vegetables, and some plants.

Stemphylium: Grows near water, on bark, cotton, canvas, damp paper, and books.

Trichoderma: Grows on decaying wood, damp cotton and wool, and in basements.

To check for molds, one places mold plates throughout the home, especially in places that look suspicious. Mold plates are plastic dishes lined with a special medium to which mold spores will automatically attach themselves. Any watermarks or discolorations on walls or ceilings probably indicate molds. Bathrooms can be notorious hiding places for molds and mildews, as can damp basements. After mold plates have been exposed for fifteen to thirty minutes, they are sent to a laboratory, which will detect and identify how many types of molds are in the home and how high the levels are.

To correct mold and bacterial growth, the following steps must be taken:

- Water leaks and seepage into the home must be eliminated. Gutters can be installed, and the foundation and exterior of the home should be sealed and waterproofed. Leaking drainpipes should be repaired. Seal tubs and sinks as well.
- Repair water-damaged materials. Scrape, plaster, and freshly paint any mildewy or moldy walls and ceilings. Remove damp carpets, and place plastic sheeting over concrete floors in basements or on porches.
- If your home tends to be moist, use a dehumidifier. Keep fans in windows in laundry rooms, kitchens, and bathrooms to eliminate moisture. Also ventilate attics, basements, and crawl spaces. Keep the humidity in your home below 50 percent.

- Clean evaporation trays and drains in dehumidifiers, air conditioners, furnaces, freezers, and refrigerators. Make sure that seals on the doors of the refrigerator are firm. Dirty air conditioners and refrigerators with drip pans can be breeding grounds for molds, whose spores then float into the air and attach themselves elsewhere.
- Regularly clean and disinfect all moist surfaces, especially shower tiles and kitchen counters.
- Do not use cold humidifiers, including ultrasonic units, as they tend to grow more mold. Steam heat prevents the growth of mold.

I often find that my mold-sensitive patients are suffering from an overgrowth or hypersensitivity to candida, a yeast fungus that usually grows in harmless amounts in the body, along mucous membranes in the mouth, digestive tract, and vagina. However, because asthmatic patients may have suffered from frequent colds and respiratory infections, they often have a history of antibiotic and steroid use. Antibiotics have now been widely acknowledged to lead to yeast overgrowth; they do so by eliminating healthy as well as unhealthy flora from the digestive tract, leaving room for yeast to grow unchecked. Steroids can lead to yeast overgrowth because they directly stimulate fungal replication and because they suppress the immune system. Patients who are sensitive to candida because of an overgrowth in their own body often then become sensitized to other fungi in the environment.

I find that by reducing candida overgrowth with judicious use of natural and prescription antifungals, some patients report improved tolerance to molds. Antifungal substances include the following:

Garlic is high in sulfur compounds, which inhibit fungal growth. Use garlic liberally in salad dressings as well as cooked vegetables. Odorless garlic capsules and liquid are also available at health food stores. One popular brand is Kyolic, which comes in capsules or liquid form.

Caprylic acid is a fatty acid that is manufactured to be released in the intestinal tract. It has been proven in many studies to reduce yeast from the digestive system within days.

Artemesia is an herb that has been shown to have powerful antifungal and antiparasitic activity.

Grapefruit seed extract, commonly known as Citricidal, comes in liquid and capsule form and is a potent antifungal substance. The liquid must be diluted in water, or it will irritate sensitive tissues in the mouth and digestive tract. A diluted solution can be used to wash fruits and vegetables that might be growing molds not visible to the naked eye.

A preparation that combines both artemesia and grapefruit seed extract is known as Artemesia Forte, from Allergy Research Group. It is a particularly effective combination.

Nystatin is an antifungal antibiotic named after New York State, where it was discovered in the soil. It is well tolerated by most individuals and is not absorbed outside the gastrointestinal tract. It can be mixed with water and used as a mouthwash or douche, as well as taken internally.

Azoles are a class of quite potent systemic antifungal drugs. These include fluconazole (Diflucan), ketaconazole (Nizoral), and itraconazole (Sporanox). These drugs can be very effective in reducing fungal overgrowth within a matter of weeks. They must also be monitored with blood tests, as this class of drugs has been shown to cause liver damage in rare cases, especially with long-term use.

In all cases where antifungal products are taken, patients must supplement their diet with yogurt that contains acidophilus and/or bifido-bacteria, as well as beneficial flora products sold in health food stores. These are friendly strains of bacteria that our bodies tolerate well and that help keep yeast in check. Refrigerated acidophilus products are the most reliable and potent; unrefrigerated products that have been sitting on the shelf for months may have lost their potency. These friendly bacteria are known as probiotics (as opposed to antibiotics). In other words, you are adding strains of bacteria to your system that are healthy for you and can help fight yeast without drugs.

You may be surprised to hear that your internal environment may be so directly linked to your external environment. In the case of molds, which are so highly allergenic in so many asthma patients, this is particularly true. I always recommend a two-pronged approach when treating mold sensitivity: first, I check to see if there is a history of antibiotic and steroid use (or for some people, a high-sugar diet) that might stimulate yeast overgrowth, and then I work to eliminate molds from the home and office.

Pests, dust mites, and dander. Many individuals are sensitive to the fecal particles and body parts of cockroaches, mice, and other rodents. Dust mites, which are invisible to the naked eye and thrive in dust and humid, warm environments, are another common allergen. Their fecal particles cling to dust, become airborne, and cause asthma and allergies. The mites feed on human skin particles and can be found in carpets, beds, linen, fabric-covered furniture and stuffed toys. If you have ever seen a picture of a dust mite (magnified many times), it looks exactly like a large beetle with a curved, helmetlike shell and pincerlike legs. In fact, it belongs to the family of eight-legged insects called arachnids, which includes spiders, ticks, and chiggers. Imagine those mites living in your bedding and pillows as permanent boarders.

Dust mites tend to peak in July and August, though levels stay high through December. They are lowest in April and May. Above five thousand feet, dust mites do not grow, and so individuals allergic to dust may do well in Denver or Santa Fe or other mountain environments. Direct sunlight has been shown to be one of the best ways to rid carpets of mites. Placing rugs upside down outdoors on a sunny, hot day will kill 100 percent of mites and mite eggs.

The dander of household pets can be a problem for many individuals as well. Products are available that cleanse the animal's skin and fur of dander and saliva. Hot-water washing is very important for eliminating dander and mites. Use washable area rugs rather than carpeting. Wash bedding and rugs in hot water every ten days to eliminate dust mites. Dust with a damp or oiled cloth, and wear a dust mask while cleaning.

Normal vacuuming will not help and can, in fact, spew allergens into the air. Nilfisk manufactures a vacuum that is used by NASA scientists and cleans up even the tiniest airborne particles and dust mites. It's expensive, but it may be a lifesaver for extremely allergic individuals. Another option is to use carpet sprays that seal in dust and dust mites. Sprays containing tannic acid kill up to 92 percent of dust mites, according to research at the University of Virginia in Charlottesville. However, a popular product containing benzyl benzoate has been shown to be ineffective.

If you want your home analyzed for dust mites or pet dander you can obtain an air filtration device that attaches to your vacuum cleaner and sucks in particles that can then be analyzed by a laboratory. This can be useful in some hard-to-diagnose cases. For instance, a patient of mine bought a used sofa and soon found that her asthma had inexplicably worsened. When we used this device and vacuumed the cushions, we discovered cat dander. It turned out that the previous owner had a cat.

THE DANGERS OF MOISTURE

Moisture can potentiate many airborne contaminants. Many people believe it's healthy to humidify their house, yet they do not understand the importance of regulating levels of humidity. There are big drawbacks to an overly moist atmosphere, and even tabletop cold-air humidifiers can breed molds that cause respiratory problems in sensitive individuals. Humidity must be carefully regulated so that moisture levels do not exceed 50 percent, and a humidified house needs to be clean of contaminants. Moisture is a catalyst for many household chemicals and allergens. Formaldehyde levels, for instance, can be elevated by heat and humidity. Dust mites multiply much more quickly at levels of humidity over 50 percent. Molds and bacteria grow far more rapidly in the presence of moisture.

You can check humidity in your environment with a simple device called a hydrometer.

Attacking trouble spots and ridding your home of toxic contaminants is a time-consuming but infinitely worthwhile approach to asthma. As a general rule, however, you should always ventilate your home or office. In the warmer months, this is easily done by opening windows and doors and installing simple ventilating fans, allowing toxins to escape on air currents. Air conditioners tend to recirculate air and are not helpful. Air filter machines can be a lifesaver.

In the winter, one option is an appliance known as a heat-recovery ventilator (HRV), which can be mounted in a wall or window just like an air conditioner. It brings fresh, filtered outdoor air into the home, while sucking out stale indoor air. These machines can cost up to fifteen hundred dollars.

Check the listing in *Resources* for a firm that manufactures excellent air filters. Certain companies, such as Austin Air, Inc., specialize in units that take care of specific toxins in work or home environments. It is my belief that Austin Air makes one of the best filters on the market: they contain far more activated carbon than most.

Homesick Syndrome Questionnaire

What follows are questions I ask my patients to determine just how much of their asthma might be triggered by a sick home or office. Because you have just read an explanation of the various hot spots and toxins in a typical sick home or building, you will understand why I ask these questions. For instance, chemicals can outgas when drapes are dry-cleaned; molds can grow on old, damp newspapers; remodeling with particleboard can be a source of formaldehyde.

1. How long have you lived in this home?
2. Does being in your home make you feel ill?
3. Do you feel ill when doors and windows are open? Closed?
4. Is a particular time of day the worst?
5. What symptoms disappear when you leave your home?
6. Have you recently purchased new carpet? Drapes? Furniture? Cabinets or bookcases? Gas appliance, furnace, or stove? Pressed board, particleboard, or plywood?
7. Have you recently dry-cleaned your drapes or clothes?
8. Have you recently changed dry-cleaners?
9. Has a service company cleaned your carpet or furniture?
10. Do you store large amounts of newspaper? Cardboard? Cleaning products? Pest-control products?
11. Do you have any pets?
12. Have you recently used cleaning solvents, wood strippers, varnish, stains, paints, or glues?
13. Have you recently performed any remodeling or repairs?
14. Have you recently used pest-control products or lawn-care products or pesticides?

Home Evaluation

The following chart details the results of a home evaluation conducted for Lisa J. in February 1992 by Ecosafe™. (If you suspect that your home is causing some of your health problems, it may be wise to have a similar evaluation.)

INTRODUCTION

In early February 1992 Ecosafe™ Environmental was contacted by Mrs. Lisa J. for the purpose of evaluating her home, located in New Jersey, for potential air- and water-quality problems. On 2/25/1992, an Ecosafe™ technician performed an indoor evaluation at the home.

Mrs. J complained that both of her children suffer from allergies. An evaluation of the indoor air and water quality was performed, as well as an evaluation of the outside environment.

A walk-through of your home revealed several areas of concern, which included the use of wall-to-wall carpeting on the entire upper floor, the usage of the humidifier, a fish tank, as well as wall-to-wall carpeting in the main playing area, and an attached indoor garage.

PURPOSE OF THE EVALUATION

The purpose of this report is to provide an assessment of potential health hazards in your home, and to document the presence or absence of suspected environmental contaminants. Recommendations for future sampling and analysis, as well as feasible mitigation techniques and remediation options are also discussed.

"Allowable Limits" for potential Health Hazards discussed in this report are those established by federal or industrial regulatory agencies, such as OSHA or NIOSH, for the workplace, schools, or commercial and public buildings.

Keep in mind that residential contaminant exposure

levels that appear to be safe for individuals because they are below OSHA and NIOSH exposure standards are very capable of causing major health problems. However, exposure levels above OSHA or NIOSH standards should be corrected immediately.

This evaluation was based upon available site history, observable conditions, as well as on-site investigation. Please note that an investigation cannot absolutely rule out the existence of any hazardous materials.

1. FUNGI SOURCE INSPECTION

There are several types of biological fungi contamination which can be found in the average home or office. They include unicellular forms, such as molds and mildew, which are by far the most common mushrooms and plant disease organisms. Some fungi are eukaryotic, like human cells, while others are multicellular, and still others are specialized for dispersal.

Biological contaminants may be the most common health problem associated with indoor air quality. They are a known health risk for individuals who are susceptible to or have known allergenic health problems. They also can become a risk to healthy individuals through exposure to higher than normal levels of contamination.

Biological contaminants can trigger many allergic reactions including asthma, pneumonitis, infections, and allergic rhinitis. Disease-causing toxins can be released by some molds and mildews. Toxins released by fungi have in some instances been found to be carcinogenic. Fungus growing on a water reservoir can be released into the air and may be a source of pneumonitis.

Symptoms of health problems associated with fungi biological pollutants include watery eyes, sneezing, coughing, urticaria, fatigue, headaches, nasal congestion, and occasionally digestive complaints. Individuals with respiratory problems and pulmonary diseases are especially at risk.

Testing for mold growth in your home was performed. Moderate mold growth was found in your den and the baby room. A description of the molds is included in the laboratory report at the end of the discussion. The predominant organism found included candida albicans, cladosporium, and alternaria.

A walk-through inspection of your home did not reveal any visual mold growth.

REMEDIATION OF FUNGAL GROWTH

All areas which may have fungal growth, such as the bathroom areas, the fish tank, or any surfaces in the den and the baby's room, should be treated with an antifungal agent, such as a solution of borax and water, or borax and white vinegar, or Zephrin. Attempts should be made to keep either a dehumidifier in the affected rooms or keep the areas as dry as possible. Special attention should be given to good ventilation. Dampness on carpeting may be remedied by sprinkling corn starch or baking soda on or over the affected areas. It is advisable to remove the carpeting in the baby room and the den.

2. LEAD

Lead is a metallic element used to make pipes, machinery, toys, paint, gasoline, pottery, and china. It is released into the air through the sanding, breakdown or burning of lead-based paint, soldering (water pipes and some metal cans), electronic repair, construction or breakage of pottery and china, and automobile exhaust.

Lead, in both high and low concentrations, is toxic to many organs within the body and may enter the body through the digestive or the respiratory tract. Lead exposure is known to permanently lower a child's IQ and cause attention disorders. Lead poisoning affects the brain, nervous, blood, and digestive systems, causing weight loss, anemia, stomach cramps, convulsions, depression, and kidney damage. Minimal lead levels may increase high blood pressure in adults.

OSHA's guideline for acceptable lead exposure is under court remand. Leading health experts have stated that there is not a safe level of lead exposure. The use of lead paint has been banned since 1978 and it is being removed from gasoline.

Although no lead was detected in the water, it is quite possible that a retest on first use in the morning might show higher levels of lead.

3. DUST MITES

Dust may contain fibers, hair, skin, molds, soot, and pollen. Dust mites and their waste products are one of the most important allergenic substances. The mite can be primarily found in mattresses, pillows, blankets, curtains, stuffed toys, carpets, and upholsteries. Symptoms associated with "house dust" are sneezing, nasal congestion, itching and running of the eyes, skin rashes, and asthma.

REMEDIATION OF DUST MITES

Your dust mite count is considered to be significant, and steps to remedy this problem are advised. First, clean the carpet and upholstery in your den with an allergy control solution. Second, consider removing the carpet. Third, it is recommended to encase mattress, boxspring, and the pillows with allergy proof coverings. And fourth, an air purifier with an HEPA filter is strongly recommended.

4. PESTICIDES

Pesticides are man-made chemical compounds used in and around a home to control plants and weeds (herbicides), insects (insecticides), termites (termiticides), rodents (rodenticides), and fungi (fungicides). They are sold as sprays, sticks, powders, crystals, balls, foggers, bombs, and liquids. In addition to the active targeted pest, they also contain an inactive carrying agent not toxic to the targeted pest, but which can be toxic to humans. Remember, the "cide" means to kill. When applied outdoors, they often will contaminate the air, soil, and water supply.

Pesticide vapors, however, are a known health risk to individuals who are susceptible to or have known health problems. Pesticide vapor exposure can also be a risk to healthy individuals. Recent studies have pointed to pesticide vapor contamination as a contributor to immune system breakdown. The health effects from exposure to pesticides include irritation to eyes, nose, throat, and skin; cancer; damage to the nervous system; liver and kidney damage; and death.

References were made concerning pesticide use around your home, by your neighbors. Efforts should be made to reduce or exclude the use of pesticides in areas where children play.

REMEDIATION OF PESTICIDES

To mitigate pesticide exposure, read the label and follow the directions on the container. It is illegal by federal law to use a pesticide in any manner that is inconsistent with directions on its label and to use a restricted pesticide.

Never apply pesticides in quantities greater than what is being called for on the product label or apply them in heating and air-conditioning duct work. Always mix or dilute pesticides in a well-ventilated outdoor area and in the recommended quantities. Use nonchemical methods of pest control when possible. A properly fertilized, watered, tended, and aerated lawn will reduce the necessity for pesticides.

Store unneeded pesticides out of the home in a secured area and keep firewood stacked away from your home to reduce termite damage. Dispose of empty, unwanted pesticide containers safely and return banned chemicals to the manufacturer.

If you employ a commercial pest control company, select it carefully and monitor their actions. Ask for a written program listing specific names of pests to be controlled and the chemicals to be used. Verify that the company and technicians are both licensed for application of pesticides, especially termiticides. Monitor their work and be sure that you receive a copy of the applied pesticide label, product safety data sheet, and diagram of where the pesticide was applied. It is advisable to let family members take their shoes off while in the home to reduce possible exposure to pesticides brought in from the outside.

5. AMMONIA AND CHLORINE

It was noted that you were using ammonia and chlorine products.

Ammonia is a colorless, soluble gas, one part nitrogen and three parts hydrogen, that has a pungent, suffocating smell, and strong alkaline reaction. It is a very common ingredient in household cleaners and used for other purposes. Ammonia exposure causes irritation of the eyes, nose, throat, and respiratory tract; eye and skin burns; and chest pains.

To mitigate ammonia exposure, always use products containing it in a well-ventilated area. Should the skin come in contact with ammonia, flush the affected area with fresh water, then immediately wash with soap. DO NOT EVER MIX AMMONIA WITH CHLORINE; THE RESULTING CHLORAMINE FUMES CAN BE DEADLY.

Chlorine is a poisonous, greenish-yellow, gaseous chemical element found in common salt. It is used for bleaching, disinfecting, and the treatment of drinking water. Exposure to chlorine causes irritation to the nose, throat, and the lungs. It also produces carcinogenic vapors when it reacts with decaying vegetation.

Decrease exposure to chlorine gas by wearing a dust mask when using products containing it and avoid using chlorine products near vegetation. DO NOT EVER MIX CHLORINE WITH AMMONIA; THE RESULTING CHLORAMINE FUMES CAN BE DEADLY.

6. CARBON MONOXIDE

Carbon monoxide is a colorless, odorless gas that is a by-product of unvented gas, leaking chimneys and furnaces, downdrafting from wood stoves and fireplaces, gas appliances, tobacco smoke, and automobile exhausts.

Carbon monoxide interferes with the uptake of oxygen throughout the body. Low concentrations can cause healthy individuals to suffer fatigue, and increase episodes of chest pain for those with chronic heart disease. Higher concentration can cause headaches, dizziness, weakness, nausea, confusion, or disorientation. Symptoms of carbon monoxide poisoning at this level are often confused with the flu or food poisoning. Very high concentrations of carbon monoxide can cause unconsciousness and death.

A walk-through inspection revealed that your garage is attached to the den where the children most likely play. Evaluation of your car showed high levels of interior carbon monoxide while the car was running. Installing an exhaust fan in the garage is recommended.

SUMMARY

Efforts should be made to clean all areas which show fungi growth in the manner as discussed. A dehumidifier should be placed in the den or the baby's room. The removal of the carpet in these rooms is recommended.

Mattress and pillows should be encased by allergy-proof coverings, to reduce exposure to mold and dust mites.

If tap water is used, it is recommended to cook the water or leave the water out for 24 hours to remove the chlorine. Water should be stored in a glass container. However, the water could be retested for possible chlorine and bacterial contamination.

A HEPA (high-efficiency particle air) filter unit is strongly recommended to reduce any airborne toxins or dust, especially in the baby's room and the playing area.

Any stuffed toys should be removed while [the baby is] sleeping.

Efforts should be made to use more natural household products.

A test for radon is recommended.

· Special thanks to RCI Environmental for their help in preparing this report.

PART 2:
OCCUPATIONAL ASTHMA

As long ago as the year A.D. 23, stone carvers covered themselves in sacks and used animal bladders as masks to protect themselves against dust—and asthma. A great Greek physician, Galen, noted that certain professions seemed to lead to asthma, and he used to send asthmatic miners, tanners, and other craftsmen up the slopes of the volcano, Mt. Etna, to inhale the therapeutic fumes of sulfur. The sulfur, which was an irritant, probably caused them to cough up mucus.

Many occupations can lead to asthma, caused by toxins and allergens spewed into the air by certain products in the course of the work process. Asthma can occur in people who work with latex, resins, dyes, metals, drugs, and insects. Aeronautical engineers may suffer from asthma due to thinners, solvents, anticorrosives, latex, formaldehyde, acrylic glues, and more. Veterinarians, pet shop owners, farmers, zookeepers, and animal breeders are known to suffer from asthma triggered by dander, feathers, saliva, and urine from animals, along with deodorants and vermifuges used around the animals. Artists can become sensitized to acrylics, resins, pigments, thinners, solvents, and polishes. Automotive body mechanics have come down with asthma triggered by brake fluid, gasoline, cleansers, chromium, anticorrosive paints, and nickel. Woodworkers, pulp workers, bark strippers, cork workers, and carpenters can be allergic to wood pulp, sawdust, tree bark, cork, and the various fungi that live on wood. Pharmacists and physicians can become allergic to antibiotics or latex gloves (10 percent of surgeons now have latex allergies). Grain handlers and bakers can be allergic to the dust in soybeans and grains.

The list for occupational asthma goes on, including documented cases of asthma in bronze workers, cable splicers, carpet makers, chemists, dairy workers, battery makers, dry cleaners, electricians, dentists, hairdressers and barbers, florists and horticulturists, jewelers, laundry workers, medical personnel, sewer workers, shoemakers, railroad workers, printers, plastics makers, textile workers, and upholsterers. Now, with the advent of sick buildings, even regular office workers are subject to occupational asthma.

Indeed, no occupation seems safe. A report from the *Journal of the American Podiatric Medical Association* noted that nearly a third of all podiatrists have IgE (allergic) antibodies to a common mold that causes toenails to become infected with fungus. The treatment is often to burn the thick, yellowed nails, a procedure that causes the doctor to inhale nail dust, 86 percent of which reaches the lungs. Podiatrists who are chronically exposed to nail dust suffer from conjunctivitis, rhinitis, asthma, coughing, and impaired lung function.

Occupational asthma often follows a very distinct pattern. Symptoms improve when a patient is away from work (on the weekend, for example) and worsen on his or her return. One of my patients, a pizza baker, had no idea he was allergic to flour dust, and spent every day pounding the dough, inhaling clouds of airborne flour.

The solutions to occupational asthma are varied. Occasionally the asthma is so severe the individual needs to alter his or her work environment or occupation. In the case of the baker who was my patient, he changed his job from pounding the dough to slicing the vegetables and cheese, and he wore a mask whenever he was near the dusty part of the kitchen.

In general, however, the answer to sick air is to clean up the air and to boost the immune system in all the ways you will discover as you read this book.

PART 3:
OUTDOOR AIR

Indoor air can be cleaned up. Outdoor air cannot—at least not on an individual level. Neither can we test the quality of outdoor air by ourselves. For most of us, there is little or no information about the quality of our air. California is one of the few states that measures and announces ozone levels every day. The rest of us wake up each morning and venture out into the world without knowing whether soot, ozone, pollens, molds, or countless other toxins have soared to levels that may precipitate an asthma attack.

Pollution has become such an accepted phenomenon that many disasters occur with little publicity. Last year I noticed a small story hidden in the back of *The New York Times* about a faulty valve in a factory in New Jersey that spewed out a cloud of toxic gas. Nearly fifty people were hospitalized with respiratory illness, but the story itself was clearly not considered major news.

Although I could list all the major pollutants in our atmosphere, it would not help you to get better. For instance, sulfur dioxide is a common pollutant (most often emitted by coal or oil-fired electric power plants) that can cause asthma attacks in concentrations of only 1 part per million.

We do not have to be entirely at the mercy of outdoor air, however. There are tools we can utilize to help guide and protect us.

Simple Rules for the City

I recently saw an asthma patient, Bill, who at thirty-four years old was a dedicated runner. He was convinced that his daily jog after work helped keep his lungs in shape and him out of the hospital, and he probably was right. Since he had begun a jogging program five years earlier, his health had improved greatly. Nonetheless, he was troubled by frequent tightness and wheezing, especially in the evenings. On a hunch, I asked him to stop jogging after work, when rush hour traffic pours exhaust into the air. I suggested he run in the early morning, when pollution levels are lowest. I also asked him not to run down congested First Avenue, but instead to limit his jogging to the reservoir around Central Park, far from the cars and buses. He noticed a difference immediately.

If you live in the city like Bill, follow simple, common-sense rules. Don't spend a lot of time walking or jogging down polluted city streets on a regular basis. Don't exercise on days when there are ozone alerts. If you are sensitive to bus fumes, seek alternative forms of transportation, such as the train or car—or car pool. For asthmatics who are particularly sensitive, there are masks that cyclists use, and scarves with carbon filters that can be worn in the winter (see page 237). Recently, New York City lost an opportunity to buy a fleet of "clean" buses with filtered exhausts. It is this kind of decision that has an impact on the health of all of us.

In traffic, seal your windows and recirculate your air. If you can afford it, ask for a custom-made air filter to be inserted in your car's ventilation system (Mercedes now installs a special air filter in all its vehicles). Don't sit in the back of a bus, where the exhaust fumes are most intense.

Pollens

Most traditional asthma books take a good, long look at pollens. Pollinating trees, flowers, grasses, and weeds have long been acknowledged by allergists to be a source of asthma attacks. In the past, it was relatively easy for a physician to narrow down the possible causes of pollen allergy, because each area has its own indigenous, native vegetation. However, because of modern technology and sophisticated irrigation techniques, it is now possible to transplant virtually any tree or plant to any place in the world.

In general, trees in the Northeast tend to pollinate in late March, April, and May. Grass starts to pollinate around Memorial Day and continues into early August. (As you might imagine, asthmatics who are sensitive to both trees and grasses may find the "lovely month of May" to be a nightmare.) Ragweed tends to pollinate in August and peaks in early September, finally dying off in October.

In the Northwest, trees begin to pollinate in April; grasses keep pollinating into September; and weeds may pollinate through November. In southern California, trees pollinate from February through December, giving asthmatics a mere month's respite. In the dry Southwest, where molds are not much of a problem, pollens are a year-long problem, as weeds and grasses pollinate almost all year.

It is extremely important to be tested for pollen allergies. A little knowledge can change your life. For instance, ragweed hardly grows in northern Michigan and northern Maine, making these places a haven for those with this type of allergy.

TREE POLLEN SEASONS

	Jan	Feb	Mar	Apr	May	Jun	Jul	Aug	Sep	Oct	Nov	Dec
DESERT SOUTHWEST INCLUDING WEST TEXAS												
OAK			■	■	■	■						
MESQUITE			■	■	■	■						
COTTONWOOD		■	■	■								
INTERMOUNTAIN REGION												
OAK					■	■						
BIRCH					■	■						
COTTONWOOD/POPLAR				■	■	■						
BOX ELDER				■	■							
NORTHEAST/CENTRAL UNITED STATES												
OAK				■	■	■						
BIRCH				■	■	■						
COTTONWOOD/POPLAR				■	■							
MAPLE/BOX ELDER			■	■	■							
PACIFIC NORTHWEST												
OAK				■	■	■						
BLACK WALNUT				■	■							
CHINESE ELM		■	■	■								
ALDER		■	■	■								
SOUTHEAST AND SOUTH CENTRAL UNITED STATES												
OAK				■	■							
BIRCH				■	■							
PECAN				■	■							
MAPLE/BOX ELDER		■	■	■	■							

GRASS POLLEN SEASONS

	Jan	Feb	Mar	Apr	May	Jun	Jul	Aug	Sep	Oct	Nov	Dec
DESERT SOUTHWEST INCLUDING WEST TEXAS												
BERMUDA					X	X	X	X	X	X		
BROME					X			X				
JUNE (KENTUCKY BLUE)					X			X				
SUDAN GRASS				X	X	X	X	X	X			
INTERMOUNTAIN REGION												
TIMOTHY					X	X	X	X				
ORCHARD					X	X	X	X				
JUNE (KENTUCKY BLUE)					X	X	X	X				
BROME					X	X	X	X				
NORTHEAST/CENTRAL UNITED STATES												
TIMOTHY					X	X	X	X				
ORCHARD					X	X	X	X				
JUNE (KENTUCKY BLUE)					X	X	X	X				
RED TOP					X	X	X	X				
PACIFIC NORTHWEST												
TIMOTHY				X	X	X	X	X				
ORCHARD				X	X	X	X	X				
ITALIAN RYE				X	X	X	X	X				
JUNE GRASS				X	X	X	X	X				
BROME				X	X	X	X	X				
SOUTHEAST AND SOUTH CENTRAL UNITED STATES												
BERMUDA		X	X	X	X	X	X	X	X	X	X	
JOHNSON					X	X	X	X	X	X		
JUNE (KENTUCKY BLUE)					X	X						
TIMOTHY					X	X						
ORCHARD					X	X						

WEED POLLEN SEASONS

	Jan	Feb	Mar	Apr	May	Jun	Jul	Aug	Sep	Oct	Nov	Dec
DESERT SOUTHWEST INCLUDING WEST TEXAS												
WESTERN RAGWEED			■	■	■	■	■	■	■	■		
FALSE RAGWEED			■	■	■	■	■					
COTTONWOOD		■	■	■	■							
INTERMOUNTAIN REGION												
WESTERN RAGWEED								■	■			
FALSE RAGWEED								■	■			
SAGEBRUSH								■	■	■		
ENGLISH PLANTAIN					■	■	■		■			
RUSSIAN THISTLE						■	■	■	■	■		
NORTHEAST/CENTRAL UNITED STATES												
SHORT RAGWEED								■	■	■		
TALL RAGWEED								■	■			
LAMB'S QUARTERS								■	■	■		
ENGLISH PLANTAIN					■	■	■					
PACIFIC NORTHWEST												
WESTERN RAGWEED						■	■		■	■		
FALSE RAGWEED						■	■					
ENGLISH PLANTAIN					■	■	■					
SOUTHEAST AND SOUTH CENTRAL UNITED STATES												
TALL RAGWEED								■	■	■		
SHORT RAGWEED								■	■	■		
LAMB'S QUARTERS								■	■	■		
ENGLISH PLANTAIN				■	■	■	■					

These charts are not intended to be a complete listing , but rather to give an idea of pollination patterns in the United States. Local variations may occur because of elevation, temperature, and rainfall.

Special thanks to Center Laboratories, Meridian Bio-Medical, Inc., and Mary Jelks, M.D. for their assistance in assembling this information.

For an asthmatic who suffers from hay fever, the spring, summer, and early fall are often hellish. In March and April, many common trees flower and their pollens sally forth on the wind. In the early summer, many grasses can cause allergies, and in late summer, ragweed blooms in a golden nightmare that can cause sleepless nights for sufferers.

If you are not certain if you suffer from pollen allergies, here are a few helpful hints:

- Pollen counts are often high in the morning.
- Pollen allergies are worse on clear and windy days.
- Allergies to pollen improve after the first frost.
- Rain tends to keep pollen out of the air and may improve your symptoms.
- Pollen allergies will improve inside in an air-conditioned environment.

Molds

Just when an asthmatic has made it through the spring and summer, along comes autumn with its increased mold counts, spurred on by damp leaves underfoot. Yet molds can flourish at any time of year—even in winter in certain warmer climates. Molds are extremely hardy and reproduce by sending out spores (similar to seeds) that are about one-tenth the size of a red blood cell. In a moldy environment, you may be inhaling millions of spores with every breath.

Outdoor molds prefer certain seasons. For instance, in the Northeast, molds grow as soon as the mercury in the thermometer rises above fifty-five degrees. Some molds, such as alternaria and hormodendrum, flourish through August. As they fall off, other molds take their place. Even after a first frost molds can grow, because as soon as it warms up, the molds grow in the wet soil and send out a rocket blast of spores. In the South, molds are practically a year-round problem. In the Pacific Northwest, molds grow almost constantly. Even in the arid desert, where you may find relief from molds, a few species of fungi flourish.

If you are not certain if outdoor molds are causing your symptoms, here are some helpful clues:

- When temperatures are below freezing, you will feel better.
- At the water's edge, in the desert, and in the mountains, molds are less likely to grow, and you will feel better at these places. Ironically, molds are less likely to grow in our polluted concrete-and-steel cities, and some mold-sensitive individuals hide out in urban meccas during spring and summer rather than risk a wonderful "vacation" in the country.
- After raking leaves, your asthma symptoms will worsen if you are mold sensitive.
- Your asthma will tend to be worse outdoors in the evening air. Molds flourish in the evening. During the day, when the sun is out, the drier, brighter environment tends to inhibit mold growth.
- You will feel worse on rainy, humid days. Mold counts tend to be highest on such days.
- You will be frustrated to find that your asthma symptoms continue beyond the ragweed season, into the autumn.

The information in this chapter may seem overwhelming to you. There are times when I myself—considering the invisible billions of mold spores, soot particles, dust mites, and countless contaminants I am inhaling with every single breath—feel a bit overwhelmed. But part of the reason I have laid out the truth in such detail here is to inspire you to clean up your environment as much as you can. Even simple changes like lowering humidity, ventilating your home, and buying an air filter can make a tremendous difference in your breathing capacity. Regularly washed linens and a mattress cover on your bed and pillow may change you from a restless sleeper with nocturnal asthma into a rested individual who sleeps soundly through the night.

After all, what is asthma all about? Breathing. Let's try to make sure the air we breathe is clean.

RESOURCES

The following organizations can provide helpful information, procedures, devices, and household products for testing and cleaning up your environment:

- Allergy Control Products, 96 Danbury Road, Ridgefield, CT 06877, 800-422-DUST. Manufacturer of many products to help reduce dust mites, from pillow and mattress covers to machine-washable stuffed animals for children to solutions that kill dust mites and/or inactivate allergy-causing substances in dust; also masks, E-Z spacer, nebulizers, and peak flow meters.
- Allergy Research Group, P.O. Box 489, 400 Preda Street, San Leandro, CA 94577-0489, 800-545-9960.
- Allergy Resources, 557 Burbank Street, Suite K, Broomfield, CO 80020, 800-USE-FLAX. A catalogue with hundreds of home products for allergy sufferers, from cotton bedding to natural cleaning products, air filters, air purifiers (ozone), shower filters, water filters.
- Allerpet, P.O. Box 2220, Lenox Hill Station, New York, NY 10021, 212-861-1134. Supplier of a product that reduces the volume of allergens contained on an animal, cleansing the fur and skin of dander and saliva.
- Alpha Energy Laboratories, 1555 Valwood Parkway, Suite 100, Carrollton, TX 75006, 972-243-0341.

- American Academy of Environmental Medicine, 10 East Randolph Street, New Hope, PA 18938. 215-862-4574, 800-LET-HEAL.
- Austin Air Systems, Buffalo, NY 14210, 800-724-8403. Makers of Healthmate™ (HEPA filter) and Healthmate Plus™ (custom-made filters).
- Benjamin Moore and Co., Paint Supplies, 51 Chestnut Ridge, Montvale, NJ 07645, 201-573-9600 or 800-826-2623. Non-toxic paints.
- Consumer Product Safety Commission, Publisher Requests, Washington, DC 20207, 800-638-2772, ext. 300.
- Department of Environmental Protection: 718-DEP-HELP (Water quality) Daily Pollen and Mold Count: 718-470-4610, Daily Ozone Level: 800-535-1345.
- E. L. Foust Co., Inc., Box 105, Elmhurst, IL 60126, 800-225-9549. Manufacturer of an air purification system that includes activated carbon filters and HEPA filters for maximum control of chemicals and particles.
- Environmental Construction Outfitters, 190 Willow Street, Bronx, NY 10454, 800-238-5008. State of the art building products, services, and technologies.
- Environmental Protection Agency (EPA), 401 M Street, S.W. Washington, DC 20460, 800-490-9198, for publication and information.
- Lab Safety Supply, P.O. Box 1368, Janesville, WI 53547, 800-356-2855. A catalogue with more protective products than you have dreamed of in your entire lifetime.
- Murco Wall Products, Inc., 300 N.E. 21st Street, Fort Worth, TX 76106, 817-626-1987. A source of healthy building products.
- Pollution Solution, 126 Chambers Street, New York, NY 10007, 800-706-5007. Air filters, water filters, vacuum cleaners.
- Priorities, 70 Walnut Street, Wellesley, MA 02181, 800-553-5398. Allergy relief products for home and environmental control.

- Real Goods, 555 Leslie Street, Ukiah, CA 95482, 800-762-7325. A source for everything from scarves with charcoal filters to cleaning solvents made of natural citrus.
- RCI Environmental, 17772 Preston Road, Suite 202, Dallas, TX 75252, 214-250-6608. Testers for environmental contaminants.
- RCI Publications, 17772 Preston Road, Suite 202, Dallas, TX 75252, 214-250-6608. *Homesick Syndrome: A Guidebook to Residential Environmental Health Hazards.*
- Sierraire by Klaire Laboratories, Inc., 1573 W. Seminole, San Marcos, CA 92069, 800-533-7255. Portable air filters.
- Terra Verde Trading Co., 120 Wooster Street, New York, NY 10012, 212-925-4533. Environmental supplies for home and office, hardware, paints, polishes, etc.
- The Old-Fashioned Milk Paint Company, Box 222, Groton, MA 01450, 508-448-6336.

DOCTOR'S RECOMMENDATIONS FOR ACTION

1. The massive increase in both indoor and outdoor pollution is a significant cause in the dramatic rise in asthma around the world. Purifying your environment can go a long way toward reducing symptoms of asthma.

2. First, address your home environment. Your home can be a source of countless contaminants, from bacteria to molds, dust, and man-made toxins.

- Take my Homesick Syndrome Questionnaire.
- Have your home evaluated for formaldehyde outgassing. If there are significant sources of formaldehyde, they need to be removed. This may mean removing new, synthetic carpeting or furniture. Check fiberboard and particleboard, which is often used under plywood or wood veneers. Replace with solid wood furniture. However, check with a professional environmental expert and your physician before making any changes.

- Purchase an air filter and/or ozone machine for rooms in your house where you spend a great deal of time, such as the bedroom or a home office. Avoid being in the room when an ozone machine is on.
- Monitor all gas appliances for carbon monoxide leakage.
- Check your home for lead dust. A professional must remove lead paint.
- If you feel worse while taking a shower, purchase a shower filter that eliminates chlorine gas. Also check the bathroom for signs of mildew.
- When painting your home, use nontoxic, natural paints.
- Check your home for molds. Any discoloration on the walls is an indication of mold. Portions of walls infested with mold may need to be removed. Mold counts can be taken by a professional. If specific molds are high, the home may need to be renovated, specially cleaned, and the humidity lowered. The home must be checked for water leakage, water-damaged materials must be repaired, evaporation trays and drains throughout the house must be cleaned, and all surfaces regularly disinfected.
- If molds are a problem in your home, make sure the humidity is below 50 percent.
- If you are sensitive to molds, you may need to check the levels of yeast/candida growth within your body. Lowering your overall load of fungus can reduce your sensitivity to molds in the environment. You can alter your diet and take antifungal preparations.
- Ask your doctor to test your allergies to dust. If you are allergic to dust, which means you are actually allergic to dust mites, you may need to replace carpeting with washable rugs. Placing rugs in the hot sun for an afternoon kills all dust mites. Special sprays can reduce dust mites. You can obtain a special device that attaches to your vacuum cleaner to collect samples for analysis. A laboratory can then determine if dust mites are a problem in your home.

- If you are allergic to pets, wash your pets frequently and use special products on both your pets as well as any rugs or fabric to keep dander from circulating in the air.

3. Once you have cleaned up your home environment, turn to your office. If you feel worse while at the office, ask your company to check heating and cooling systems. Make sure you do not work near photocopy or other ozone-emitting machines. Try to work near an open window.

4. To avoid outdoor pollution, try to follow simple, commonsense rules. Don't spend a lot of time jogging or walking down polluted city streets. Don't exercise on days when there are ozone alerts. Buy masks or scarves with carbon filters.

5. To handle allergies to pollen, first be aware of which trees pollinate during which months in your area. In March and April, for instance, many common trees flower; in early summer, many grasses cause allergies; and in late summer, ragweed and other weeds can cause severe reactions. Pollen allergies are worst in the morning, on clear and windy days, and before the first frost of autumn. On these days, you may want to try to stay inside in a filtered environment; if you must go out, be sure to carry your inhaler with you in case of an asthma attack.

6. To handle allergies to outdoor molds, know that molds flourish in the evening and in the damp. During bright, dry days, they are reduced. Molds are less prevalent at the seashore and in the desert and mountains. Mold counts are highest on rainy, humid days. Try to stay indoors in a filtered, clean environment on such days. If you venture outside, prepare yourself by taking extra antihistamines and vitamin C, and make sure you have your inhaler with you.

7. The Firshein Center offers a resource catalog of products that are specifically designed for people with allergies and asthma. For information, call 1-800-268-4692.

CHAPTER TEN

The Art of Breathing

The night I nearly died of asthma in the hospital, my heart was thundering so rapidly and my chest muscles were so fatigued that each breath was a massive effort. With the ingenuity of a desperate man, I devised one of the most important breathing exercises for asthma. As I have since discovered, it's one that is the basis of ancient yogic breathing techniques and has been applied to contemporary scientific research in breathing and relaxation. I now teach this technique to my patients along with a complete program of breathing exercises.

Sitting up in the hospital bed, acutely ill, I was determined to find a way to keep breathing through the night. The technique I devised would help me through numerous attacks over the coming year, and it now helps my patients as well.

I began by checking my pulse and counting the number of beats per minute. Because my heart was skidding along at such a mad rate, I inhaled every seven beats and exhaled for nine. This seemed to allow me to force out more air than I was taking in. I observed myself relaxing into a kind of hypnotic trance. I kept my hands on my stomach, making sure that my hands were moving up and down as I breathed, proving that I was breathing in and out with my diaphragm. By the time morning came, I had made it through the worst of the attack. I had also made a discovery: if I could concentrate on my breathing, I could not only help break an attack, I could slow my pulse and the accompanying anxiety as well. As I mentioned, I have since discovered that yogis use a similar technique to regulate their respiration.

Two of the most powerful forces in your body are your breathing and your heart rate. As you synchronize the two, you begin to lose the sensation of shortness of breath. You begin to sense the rhythms, or waves, of your own respiration, your own internal ebb and flow. Some patients who practice this type of breathing claim they get into a boundless, expanded, meditative state.

Surprising as it sounds, breath training has permanently banished asthma in some patients and has significantly helped almost every asthma sufferer who has regularly applied the technique. Unfortunately, although even the National Lung Association admits the helpfulness of breathing exercises and recommends them, most physicians do not mention them to asthma patients, and most patients don't practice breathing exercises.

A few of my patients have found that certain breathing techniques can be used instead of sprays to break an acute attack. Breathing exercises can strengthen peripheral and accessory muscles that assist you in breathing. Just like weight training, these techniques make you stronger. Most of us do not use our lungs at full capacity when breathing. There is an unused reserve of about 20 percent. In a sense, these breathing exercises are like an at-home endurance sport that trains your muscles so that you can draw in that extra 20 percent of air. That air supply can be crucial in case of an acute attack or emergency. Just as important, if you maintain the aerobic tone of your chest muscles, they will not fatigue as rapidly during an attack. You can avoid hospitalization, intubation, and intravenous medication. You can be a far healthier individual.

Best of all, these techniques give asthmatics a safety net no matter where they are or how bad an acute attack might be. After that night in the hospital, I was never quite as afraid again, and as any asthmatic knows, the acute sense of helplessness and fear that accompanies an attack can be as bad as the inability to breathe.

I recently treated a fifty-five-year-old accountant, Mark. Fair-skinned and shy, he worked in a medical center, and his office had been moved to a basement area where ventilation was poor and molds were a problem. His asthma had gotten so much worse that he was taking 100 milligrams of prednisone daily, along with inhalers and theophylline. He had a nervous temperament to begin with, but by the time he came to visit me, he was in a state of virtual panic. He had been suffering sudden attacks in the office and had been hospitalized once in the past month. Mark was very concerned because he needed his job, and yet his health was deteriorating rapidly. Worst of all, he told me, was the anxiety he felt about his sudden attacks.

"I feel helpless," he said. "I wanted to start a new career. I was going to take courses in the spring to be a medical assistant. but I'm too insecure about my health now."

The first step I took was to teach him breathing exercises. We also later analyzed the mold counts in his office, began to reduce his intake of medications, and put him on CAP. The breathing exercises, however, gave Mark relief within a week. His asthma was far from cured, but once he had learned that he could make it through an attack and control his panic with breathing and relaxation techniques, he was well on his way to recovery.

Another patient of mine works for an advertising agency in a "sick" building in New York City. Maggie is not the first patient from that building who has visited me because of health problems. In Maggie's case, her asthma was so debilitating that she felt it had shaped her entire life and held her back at major turning points. She had suffered attacks almost every week and had been on one medication or another for the last decade. She also came down with bronchitis frequently. Perhaps the greatest impact of her asthma, though, was the emotional havoc it had caused in her life. She was afraid to travel, afraid to engage in sports, and most of all, afraid to have a child because she never felt well enough. When she came to see me, she had been suffering from bronchitis for six weeks.

Maggie learned some of the more forceful breathing exercises in this chapter (in particular, The Bellows) and practiced them almost religiously. I have rarely seen a patient apply these exercises as devotedly as Maggie did—ten minutes each hour, no matter where she was. We placed her on the CAP program, and she kept up her regimen faithfully for three months. By that time, her bronchitis had disappeared. Another six months, and her asthma was markedly improved. Best of all, she felt a new confidence in her body and her ability to navigate her own illness.

Another patient, a nurse, had either been intubated or medicated with virtually every hospitalization. Once she learned the breathing exercises, she used them during an attack. Instead of panicking, she began to breathe and walked very slowly over to the emergency room and received Ventolin on a nebulizer. She was fine, and she had been given no epinephrine or cortisone, nor had she required intubation, which had always been a mainstay of her emergency treatment in the past.

Today I teach breathing exercises to my patients based on a combination of techniques from yogic traditions, from my own experience, and in particular, from the bestselling book, *How I Became a Former Asthmatic*, by well-known actor Paul Sorvino.

Sorvino successfully treated his own and his son's debilitating asthma with daily breathing exercises, some of which will be detailed in this chapter. If you want to know how effective breathing exercises can be, ask Paul Sorvino, who is founder of the Sorvino Asthma Foundation and, in the spring of 1995, was presented a special award for his work on breathing by Cornell University Medical School. A videotape demonstrating his exercises is available from the Sorvino Asthma Foundation. His book documents many cases where proper breathing techniques alleviated asthma symptoms. It also tells about a galvanizing personal experience:

> The first time my son got an asthma attack, he was four. I was holding him, and his eyes rolled back in his head. I started to drive to the doctor. I thought he'd die right in my lap. The doctor gave him a shot of adrenaline and nothing happened. Zero. Fifteen minutes later he got another shot that finally took effect. That night he worsened. I was determined never to let this happen again. My wife and I would sit at home with him after that and make him do breathing exercises every half-hour. He's a big, strapping kid now. He learned his exercises and did them, and to this day if he doesn't do his exercises, he will get an attack.

My breathing classes are three hours long and take place in the evening. Classes are limited to twelve patients, and each person is taught individually how to breathe. Invariably I will look around the room as we begin, noting the hunched and strained posture of most patients. They sit with their arms close to their bodies and their shoulders bowed in, or they assume just the opposite posture: ramrod straight as if trying to prove to the world that they are not suffering shortness of breath. Most patients, when they come for their first class, tend to look pale, tense, and tired. Over the course of the evening, I see a remarkable shift—

from shallow "shoulder" breathing to deep, diaphragmatic breathing. Their faces and bodies seem to relax. Their faces are suffused with color, and even their mouths seem fuller and looser. Such is the power of oxygen, the spark of life.

The art of breathing has been taught for thousands of years, but it is only recently that breathing techniques have begun to catch the attention of researchers, medical practitioners, psychologists, and psychotherapists. Clinical evidence shows that proper breathing can dramatically improve conditions ranging from asthma to heart disease.

How can something as simple as the way you breathe alter your well-being so profoundly? One simple reason may be that proper breathing actually signals the nervous system to relax, while shallow, spasmodic breathing signals just the opposite—alarm and danger.

The nervous system has two branches. The parasympathetic branch quiets us down and is associated with relaxation and sleep. The sympathetic branch rouses us to action and prepares us for any outside threat. The sympathetic branch triggers the "fight-or-flight" response, which is associated with shallow, rapid breathing, the sudden release of stimulants like adrenaline, increased heart rate and blood pressure, and tensed muscles ready to combat danger. A condition like asthma can lead to a life of constant fight-or-flight breathing, and therefore a continual state of arousal and stress. Eventually the body enters a state of chronic exhaustion.

This kind of breathing is a form of hyperventilation that leads to constant hypoxia, or a low oxygen level in the cells and bloodstream, according to Robert Fried, Ph.D., professor of psychology at Hunter College in New York, head of the Respiratory Psychophysiology Laboratory at Hunter College, and director of the Stress and Biofeedback Clinic at the Institute for Rational-Emotive Therapy in New York. Oxygen deprivation has an immediate, harmful effect on the brain as well—not only on cognition but on mood. Low levels of oxygen in the brain have been associated with dizziness, faintness, disorientation, vertigo, and panic attacks.

During an asthma attack, every breath is so difficult, you can't escape the mere fact and difficulty of breathing. If the attack is particularly bad and hard to break, you fear you may get too tired to breathe at all. The feel is not dissimilar to the last few miles of a marathon, when you feel you just can't make it a step farther. Like a runner's trembling thighs and calves, the muscles in an asthmatic's diaphragm cry out with exhaustion. Dr. Fried has found that a host of disorders—including asthma—can be improved by learning diaphragmatic, or deep, breathing.

Other researchers have also demonstrated the power of proper breathing. A method of relaxation called "respiration feedback"—a form of biofeedback that uses the breath to help the client achieve a state of deep relaxation—is utilized by medical practitioners here and in Europe. I use it and find it effective. It utilizes a sophisticated system that has been approved by the FDA for treatment of asthma, as well as for pain, anxiety, addiction, and tension. A machine actually feeds back sound and light signals directed by the patient's own breathing. The patient lies quietly and comfortably on his back while an infrared sensor is positioned over the upper abdomen to detect even the smallest sign of proper, diaphragmatic breathing. A headset is placed over the eyes and ears to block out noise and light. Soft sound and light are synchronized so that they increase and decrease in rhythm with the patient's inhalation and exhalation. The device has been tested here and in Europe in over twenty-four clinical studies with nearly seven hundred patients, and relaxation is achieved by most clients within four 30-minute sessions.

A similar device for consumers, for which the manufacturer makes no medical claims, is called the Breathwork Explorer. It costs about $350 and calibrates ten breath-pacing programs to the client's actual breathing. Equipped with a soft, wraparound mask containing goggles, built-in earphones, and a breath sensor, the unit allows the user to achieve advanced breathing techniques and deep relaxation with relative ease. Offered by Tools for Exploration (800-456-9887), this unit can be helpful for those asthmatics who have difficulty learning diaphragmatic breathing on their own.

How do you know if you are breathing correctly?

Take a look in the mirror. Watch yourself breathe in. Do your chest and shoulders lift? Does your upper body stiffen? Do you inhale deeply, or is your breathing shallow and limited to the upper part of your lungs? How much air are you really getting with each breath? Count your breaths. Do you breathe more than fourteen times a minute? If so, your breathing is probably too rapid and shallow. Normal breathing averages about twelve breaths a minute; diaphragmatic breathing, however, can be as slow as three or four breaths a minute.

Proper breathing is not as simple as you might think. Professional musicians and singers spend countless hours training themselves how to breathe properly. The sheathe of muscles in the diaphragm is designed like a bellows that helps the lungs expand and contract fully with each inhalation and exhalation. In chronic asthma, this muscle is exhausted and in spasm much of the time. This causes us to try to compensate, using upper-airway "accessory" muscles to breathe, muscles known as the sternocleidomastoid and trapezius. We even attempt to use our shoulders to assist our lungs. With each breath, we seem to shrug. Breathing becomes shallow and spasmodic, and the lungs never expand or contract fully. An asthmatic's lungs contain much "dead" space because of mucus plugs that trap air in the alveoli, the millions of minuscule sacs that absorb oxygen and expel carbon dioxide.

Shallow breathing is not limited to asthmatics. Drs. Gay and Kathlyn Hendricks, psychotherapists, are a husband and wife team who use breathing, posture, and movement techniques with their clients. They have taught belly, or diaphragmatic, breathing for years.

"When we first began to distinguish between Fight-or-Flight and Centered Breathing," write the Hendricks in their recent book, *At the Speed of Life*, "we were profoundly amazed at how much of the former we saw. . . . We began paying attention to breathing as we waited in line at the grocery store or sat in a subway train. Most people were locked in fight-or-flight breathing."

A 1995 study found that asthma could be induced in non-asthmatics, simply by instructing them *not* to breathe deeply when exposed to airborne irritants. Researchers found that asthmatics usually react to allergens by contracting their breathing passages instead of opening them.

Imagine an empty balloon, most of which is held in someone's tight fist. Try to blow up the balloon, and you'll only be able to inflate the neck. Now imagine that fist as your diaphragm muscles in a spasm. If you can open the fist into a relaxed hand, you can blow up the entire balloon. Your lungs can fill with life-giving oxygen, and because the richest blood flow in the lungs is at the bottom (where they are the largest), you will be flooding your body with energy.

Once patients experience the power of proper breathing, they have a tool that will last a lifetime. In fact, breathing exercises have helped asthmatics who are professional athletes. One helpful hint to keep in mind is: Focus on exhalation. According to Ian Jackson—a triathlete, fitness trainer, and author of *The Breathplay Approach to Whole Life Fitness*—if you focus on exhalation and make it the active part of the breathing process, you are essentially forcing out all old air and then letting the lungs fill naturally with fresh air. Alexi Grewal, a 1984 gold medalist in cycling, used breathing techniques to help him succeed in spite of asthma. Jackie Joyner-Kersee, a gold medalist who is considered by many to be the world's finest female athlete, has asthma.

This chapter contains breathing exercises that should be practiced daily, though some of my patients practice them as often as five or ten minutes every hour at first.

Within a few days of practicing these exercises, you should feel a change for the positive. However, to make sure you are improving your breathing capacity, monitor your progress with your peak flow meter. You may even want to make a chart and mark changes. Over a period of a few months, you'll be surprised and pleased to see how much your breathing capacity has increased.

BREATHING EXERCISES: A PACING PROGRAM

Note: If, during any of these exercises, you begin to feel lightheaded, relax and breathe normally for a minute before resuming the exercise. Sometimes when the body first receives extra oxygen during belly breathing, the response can be a feeling of lightheadedness. It's a sign that you are breathing properly!

1. Getting to Know Your Belly

One of the simplest and most common belly breathing exercises uses a book. Lie down on a mat or blanket on the floor, so that you feel comfortable. Keep your legs slightly apart. Place a hardcover book on your stomach, with the binding just touching the bottom curve of your ribcage.

Breathe in through your nose, unless you find it difficult to do so because of a cold or chronic sinusitis. Yet, while breathing through your nose, imagine that you are actually drawing air in from the back of your throat, not just your

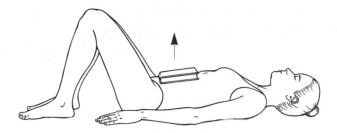

nostrils. You will notice a distinctly different sensation when you breathe this way, as if you were drawing air from some internal source. As you inhale, try to lift the book as high as you can with your stomach muscles. At the same time, try to keep your chest muscles relaxed and motionless.

Imagine that you are filling your belly with oxygen, which is then flowing from your stomach up through your chest. Your chest will expand somewhat toward the end of your inhalation.

As you exhale, use the same belly muscles to squeeze every last drop of air out of your lungs. Your exhalation should be longer than your inhalation. As you try to completely and fully contract your diaphragm muscles and push out air, the book will lower. When you've nearly reached the end of your breath, begin to hum. You will notice that even though you think you are out of air, you still have enough air left to hum for several more heartbeats.

Do this exercise slowly, so that you take about four full breaths per minute.

2. Simple Belly Breathing

Once you master the breathing technique above, you can remove the book and try the following variations on the theme:

- Lie on your back with your knees raised, feet about eight inches apart on the floor, and rock gently on your coccyx, the bone at the base of the spine. You can use an exercise mat or blanket for comfort. Rock in rhythm with your breathing, so that you arch your back off the floor slightly as you inhale, and roll your back into the floor as you exhale.

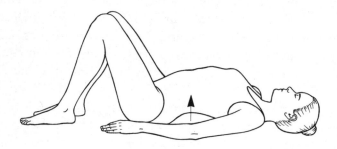

- Lie on your back as above. Swing your knees to your chest as you inhale, and then lower them back to the starting position when you exhale.

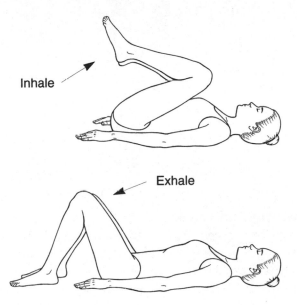

- Sit in a comfortable chair. Let your whole body relax. Place both hands palms down on your sides so that the index fingers of your hands are up against the lower ribs in the front, and your thumbs are in the back. Feel your hands move forward as you inhale, and return to their original position when you exhale. This exercise is easy to do at the office.

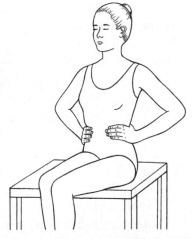

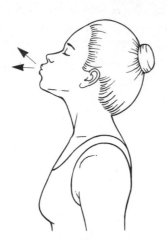

3. Blowing Out the Candle

This exercise is recommended by Paul Sorvino. It may be done sitting, standing, or lying down. Draw in a belly breath. Upon exhalation, purse your lips firmly and exhale as forcefully as you can, as if you were blowing out candles on a birthday cake. By pursing your lips this way, you produce a controlled, powerful stream of air. It will sound a bit like a speeding train.

4. Shoulder Drop

Many asthmatics tense their shoulders constantly, holding them high as if frozen in a permanent shrug. To relax chronically tense, lifted shoulders, try this exercise. Stand with your feet about twelve inches apart, letting your arms dangle freely. Bend your head forward as far as possible to stretch the back of your neck. Inhale vigorously while letting the belly distend and stick out. Swing your arms freely to the right and then the left as you inhale. Make sure your shoulders are relaxed.

Exhale a belly breath. Inhale a belly breath.

Then, on exhalation, lower your shoulders. Bring your

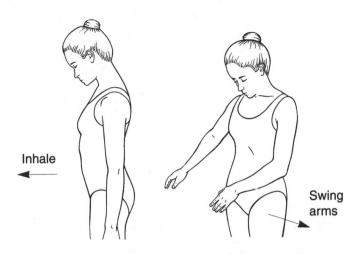

Inhale

Swing arms

head upward, and gently tilt it back as far as is comfortable, so that the front of your neck is stretched and your spine is straight. You should be exhaling forcefully through pursed lips while sucking in the lower abdomen. Swing your arms freely to the left and right as you exhale.

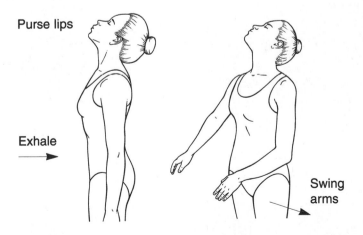

Purse lips

Exhale

Swing arms

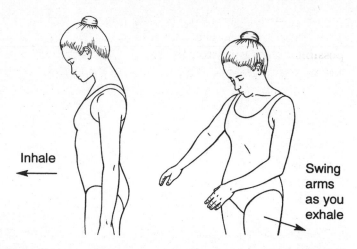

On your next breath, bend your head forward as far as is comfortable to stretch the back of your neck. Inhale a belly breath, swinging your arms to the right and left as you exhale.

5. Chest Stretch
Stand straight with your feet about ten inches apart. Lower and relax your shoulders. Shake your arms to relax yourself

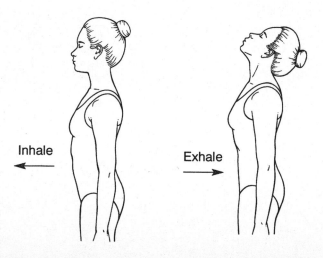

further. Let your hands dangle at your sides. Now inhale. Then exhale. As you exhale, stretch your head back as far as possible, while your stomach slowly deflates. As you inhale again, straighten up. Repeat this exercise. This will help open up the entire chest, expanding and relaxing the lungs and diaphragm.

6. Breathing Through

Drs. Gay and Kathlyn Hendricks have dubbed this technique "Presencing through Breathing." Whenever you have a strong emotion, such as panic, fear, or anger, you will shift into fight-or-flight breathing. This is especially true when an asthma attack is beginning. A cascade of physical and emotional reactions is set off. When this begins to happen, shift into belly breathing and breathe *into* the feelings. Notice your tense jaw, shoulders, chest, and neck—and any other part of your body that is in spasm. Let them relax. Let the feelings ebb and flow. You may find yourself crying or laughing, but just keep breathing with the feelings, not stopping them with short, shallow breaths or tense muscles.

Once you learn to breathe through, you will notice that the asthma attack as well as the emotions begin to subside.

7. The Bellows

This exercise is a favorite of Paul Sorvino's. Somewhat advanced, it may take time to work up to. It strengthens the diaphragm muscle itself and can dramatically lessen your susceptibility to asthma attacks.

Sit in a chair and prepare to do belly breathing. Breathe in. Start to breathe out. As you exhale, start leaning forward from the waist slowly. Pull in your diaphragm muscles as you do so. Continue to exhale as you bend forward and pull in your muscles, so that by the end of the exhalation your head is close to your knees. Now purse your lips so that you make a hissing sound as you pull your diaphragm in even tighter and exhale every last particle of air. Now begin to

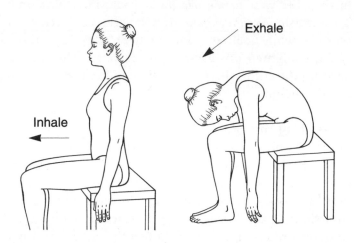

take a belly breath, inhaling slowly, and rising from the waist so that by the time you are sitting up again your lungs are filled with fresh oxygen.

Now lean forward again as quickly as you can, in a jack-knife motion, and as you do so suck in your diaphragm as if you've just been punched. Keep your lips pursed. The air should escape powerfully. When you feel you are at the end of your exhalation, repeat the hissing sound as above, until your lungs are empty. Relax, sit up slowly, and breathe in.

Even one round of bellows breathing will fill your body with fresh, restorative oxygen. You will feel more relaxed. Best of all, this exercise strengthens your diaphragm muscles so that over time they will become far more powerful and efficient.

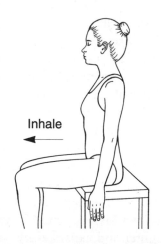

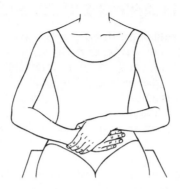

8. Heart Breathing

This final exercise is perhaps the most important of all. It is the technique I developed in the hospital and is both simple and marvelously effective. Place one hand on your stomach. Place the thumb of the other hand on the pulse of the hand resting on your stomach. Let yourself relax. Now synchronize your breathing with your heart rate. For every seven beats, breathe in. For every nine beats, breathe out. Blow out through pursed lips until your air is gone. Let your body feel the rhythm of breath and heart.

CLEARING EXERCISES

Sometimes breathing can be greatly eased by expelling mucus plugs. This can be done by lying in certain positions that drain mucus and then intentionally coughing every two or three minutes. The process can be augmented by a tried-and-true technique called "cupping," where another person thumps you on the back and shoulders. (Sometimes, thumping your chest yourself helps, too.)

Before beginning these clearing exercises, drink something hot like tea, hot milk, coffee, or hot water with lemon and honey. You can also warm and humidify the lungs by inhaling steam from the shower. This will help loosen up mucus plugs.

Position A. Lie facedown with your hips raised about twenty inches on a stack of pillows. Cough every few minutes.

Position B. Lie on your left side with your hips raised about twenty inches on a stack of pillows. Cough every few minutes.

Position C. Lie on your back with your hips raised about twenty inches on a stack of pillows. Cough every few minutes.

Position D. Lie on your right side with your hips raised about twenty inches on a stack of pillows. Cough every few minutes.

Each position helps drain a different portion of the lungs. You may find that one position tends to work best for you, or that varying the positions is most effective. This will depend on the location and severity of mucus plugs in your lungs.

One additional treatment comes from Dr. Henry Heimlich, known for his world-famous Heimlich maneuver for choking victims. He is currently studying the application of this technique for helping asthma sufferers. The Heimlich maneuver has been found to stop asthma attacks by expelling trapped air from the lungs and with it, mucus plugs. He suggests that asthma attacks may be prevented by performing the Heimlich maneuver prophylactically, thereby keeping the lungs free of mucus. Three Heimlich maneuvers are performed once a day either by another person or by the patient himself.

As he describes it: "Asthmatics continue to inhale but cannot exhale because spasm of the bronchial tubes causes blockage. The Heimlich maneuver expels the air until the asthma attack is over." And in the same article he states, "Heavy use of one of the most common inhaled asthma drugs greatly increases the risk of dying from asthma, according to new research in the February 20, 1992 issue of the *New England Journal of Medicine*. All drugs have side effects and, after a while, the patient builds up resistance to them. The Heimlich maneuver can eliminate some medication and save lives. To perform the Heimlich maneuver let the patient start breathing out, then gently use the Heimlich maneuver to expel remaining air. Repeat this after each inhalation until the asthmatic attack is over."

If you would like to try the self-administered Heimlich maneuver you must initially practice it under your physician's observation to ensure that the technique is correctly understood.

Method: Make a fist. Place the thumb side of the fist on the midline of your abdomen, halfway between bottom tip of the sternum and your navel. (*Never press against the ribs.*) Grasp your fist with your other hand. Breathe normally. Press the fist into your abdomen with quick upward pressure. The subject should experience exhalation of air and may cough up mucus. Repeat the process twice more. Should abdominal discomfort occur and persist, see a physician immediately.

This exercise, as with The Bellows exercise, is not for anyone who has experienced the following: recent surgery (particularly abdominal surgery), ulcers, hernias (particularly diaphragmatic hernias), artificial heart valves, ongoing abdominal discomfort (see physician), or pre-existing aneurysm.

For more information on the proper way to do the Heimlich maneuver on adults, infants, or on yourself, write to the Heimlich Institute (see appendix for address).

In sum, breathing is a grossly overlooked and undervalued step in treating asthma. Anyone who suffers with a respiratory condition can vastly improve his or her health by learning proper breathing techniques. Remember, breath is the first and most important way our body gets adequate oxygen levels, and breathing properly is absolutely essential for an asthmatic. Breath can indeed be life itself.

DOCTOR'S RECOMMENDATIONS FOR ACTION

1. Breathing techniques, which have been taught for thousands of years, are once again gaining popularity. Clinical evidence shows that proper breathing can dramatically improve asthma. Make breathing exercises part of your CAP program!

2. Notice whether you are breathing with shallow, rapid breaths from your upper chest, or whether you breathe deeply from your belly. Most people breathe shallowly. If you are one of those people, begin to practice breathing exercises daily.

3. Practice your breathing exercises as often as you can. I recommend a minimum of thirty minutes daily. (This can be divided up into smaller sessions.)

4. Children can take special pleasure in breathing exercises when done as a game. They can be especially beneficial when begun early.

5. Tapes on breathing exercises and visualization that I have developed can be obtained by calling my office at 1-800-268-4692.

CHAPTER ELEVEN

A Lifetime Exercise Program

If breath is life, and breathing properly is a mainstay of asthma treatment, then exercise is breath in action. I regard breathing and exercise as so closely allied that it's hard to think of one without the other. My CAP program trains patients in breathing techniques and then incorporates them into a unique exercise program. This program has a special component to it. I incorporate what is known as "pulsed" exercise: brief, intense spurts of exercise that seem to stimulate the immune system and help combat some chronic illnesses.

In addition, my exercise program incorporates breathing techniques, both those described in chapter 10 and some specific techniques to be used while exercising.

Asthma runs in my family; my father has suffered from it, as well as my mother's brother. Not surprisingly, I grew up hearing stories of asthma in "the old days." In my parents' time, an asthmatic was treated much like an invalid—kept at home, chest swathed in towels or cloths—the proverbial child with nose pressed to the windowpane, staring out at the other children tumbling, running, laughing, and playing.

By the time I was growing up, the philosophy that an asthmatic needed to spend his or her life "sitting still" had become outmoded. I played outdoors and joined in sports. In fact, my family encouraged me to lead as active a life as possible. I used to make my teammates in high school laugh because I'd run off the basketball court to take a few puffs from my inhaler, and then run back onto court, ready for the game. Looking back, it was a dangerous activity—one that's still going on among many teens today.

Even though attitudes toward asthma and exercise have changed radically in the last few decades, there is still a great deal of ignorance and misunderstanding about the subject. Many asthmatics feel so weak and fatigued and suffer so often from colds and bronchitis, that they rarely find the time or energy to begin an exercise program. Because exercise-induced asthma is so commonplace, some asthmatics become almost phobic about exercise, avoiding it at all costs. They associate exercise with the pain and terror of asthma attacks, or they feel embarrassed by the labored sound of their wheezing when they work out. "People stare at me in the gym because I make so much noise wheezing when I'm exercising," patients tell me.

Maintaining aerobic fitness helps ensure mental and physical health in very dramatic and specific ways. Exercise oxygenates the body, conditions the heart and lungs, and has helped many asthmatics keep symptoms at bay permanently. Studies conducted at the Pulmonary Function Laboratory at New York University's School of Medicine have shown that exercise can improve lung function and, within a few months, reduce exercise-induced asthma.

Asthma is a condition that can be highly variable; it can be triggered by temperature, exercise, allergies, illness, and more. Nonetheless, many people with asthma can exercise comfortably. Consider the fact that many Olympic winners and professional athletes suffer from asthma, and some of them almost died of the illness as children. At each Olympic competition, a significant number of medals are won by athletes with asthma. In the 1988 Summer Olympics, for instance, the United States won ninety-four medals, sixteen of them won by asthmatics. About 10 percent of our Olympic team is asthmatic.

As I have stated many times in this book, asthma is a disorder of the immune system, and exercise can help modulate and increase immunity.

As America becomes a fitness-conscious country, science's fascination with the impact of exercise on health has risen. Why does exercise improve health and well-being? Why, in particular, is exercise protective—sometimes extraordinarily protective—against many of the twentieth-century killers, from cancer and heart disease to diabetes, hypertension, and osteoporosis? For instance, the impact of regular exercise on cancer has been extensively researched. One 1989 study in *The American Journal of Public Health* found a remarkable link between self-reported exercise and cancer risk: relative risk of any type of cancer was 80 percent higher in inactive men, and 30 percent higher in inactive women, than in their active, exercising counterparts. If exercise can help combat the major killers of our time, surely it can improve asthma.

One patient of mine is a thirty-four-year-old banker who found that jogging really cleared out her lungs and helped her expel mucus plugs. In winter's bad weather, she wasn't able to run outside, and her asthma almost immediately worsened.

"I feel tight, I feel like I can't get a good breath," she'd complain. "I don't feel right, I can't concentrate as well at work."

These so-called "soft signs" of asthma—compared to the "hard signs" of peak-flow-meter numbers or an outright attack—are important. They indicate the quality of life.

Another patient of mine, a forty-five-year-old dentist,

had a long history of asthma. When he first came to see me, he told me he had a lot of problems trying to exercise. However, he soon began a karate and kung fu exercise program, which involves both exercise and meditation, as well as producing a lot of forceful air. When you make a kick, for instance, you exclaim loudly. At the end of that motion, you need to draw in a deep breath before you continue. Therefore, karate and kung fu teach you how to breathe, strengthen muscles and endurance, and provide good aerobic exercise. This type of exercise program helped him get off cortisone.

If all this is not enough to inspire you, consider the following, startling discoveries about the connection between exercise and health.

EXERCISE AND IMMUNITY: NEW FINDINGS

Do you wonder what is happening inside your body when you exercise and feel better? Where does that sense of well-being, clarity, and lightness come from? Why do you sleep better, handle stress more efficiently, and find that you have increased energy?

We know that moderate, sustained exercise has a positive impact on the whole immune cascade, from stress hormones to the cells that fight infection to inflammation itself. (Interestingly, sustained, extreme exercise, such as that engaged in by Olympic athletes or marathoners, can lead to a temporary decrease in resistance to upper respiratory infections. This effect has been noted for years. Heavy training can nearly double the rate of infection.) Science now has some striking and exciting new answers to our questions about exercise and immunity.

Exercise causes a dramatic increase in leukocytes (a generic name for many different types of immune cells). The number of circulating leukocytes increases up to four times during exercise and can remain elevated for up to twenty-four hours. The more intense and long-lasting the exercise, the higher the increase. For instance, less than an hour of exercise doubles leukocytes, while more than two hours quadruples levels. In trained runners, leukocytes soar from a resting level of 5.4 to an astonishing 13.7 during a three-hour treadmill run.

Exercises seem to lure T-cells, an important arm of the immune system, into circulation. The number of circulating T-cells increases up to 150 percent following exercise, although normal levels resume soon after resting. Even more interesting is the fact that regular exercise seems to alter the ratio of two types of T-cells, the T-helper and the T-suppressor. The T-helper cell is known for stimulating the body's defenses against infection, while the T-suppressor shuts down the fight. Both are involved in combating infection and work together synergistically.

In allergies, asthma, and other immune disorders, there is often an imbalance in the T-cell ratio. There are too many T-helper cells initiating the inflammatory cascade and not enough T-suppressor cells to calm the body down and return it to a resting state. Exercise can alter the ratio in favor of T-suppressor cells by as much as 50 percent. Although this change is transient (only about two hours), it's possible that over the long term, regular exercise may help by giving the body a "rest" every day.

Other branches of the immune system are also strongly impacted by exercise. For instance, B-cells are part of the so-called "humoral" immune system, which is important in producing antibodies to fight infection. The number of B-cells increases dramatically during exercise and returns to normal levels afterward. Profound alterations in killer cells are seen—with increases of up to 300 percent following exercise sessions, even sessions under thirty minutes. Killer cells return to normal levels within twenty-four hours.

Neutrophils, immune cells that fight infection, are stimulated by exercise. Even more interesting, their ability to kill bacteria seems to be enhanced by regular, moderate exercise.

Regular exercise alters stress hormones. For instance, regular training lowers levels of epinephrine and cortisol, two fight-or-flight chemicals that are released in response to stress and danger. Cytokines, substances that influence nearly all immune functions and help stimulate the growth of many different types of immune cells, are profoundly altered by exercise. Some of the most common cytokines—the interleukins—are increased by exercise. These cytokines are intimately involved in resistance to viral infection, as well as tumors.

Many significant hormones are released during exercise, and they may alter one's physical and mental well-being over time. Those hormones include ACTH, beta-endorphins, prolactin, growth hormone, thyroxine, and cortisol. In particular, regular exercise seems to increase the release of the immunostimulatory hormones (growth hormone and beta-endorphin). In fact, I know of no drug that has such a powerful stimulant effect on the immune system.

THE "EXERCISE HIGH"

Anyone who exercises has heard of and perhaps experienced the bliss of the exercise high, when the body apparently releases a flood of feel-good chemicals called endorphins. This high has been described by great athletes as "floating," "flowing," "feeling a sense of timelessness and effortlessness." Back in 1981, a fascinating study of fifteen volunteer runners was conducted at Butler Hospital in Providence. The study tested a drug called naloxone, which blocks the body's receptors for opiates, including endorphins. Dr. Richard Haier, director of the study, found that runners given naloxone experienced pain sooner than those given placebos.

Dr. Lewis Maharam, author of *The Exercise High*, feels there may be other aspects to the exercise high. When he was in high school, training for the position of pool director, he found himself one night "long past my second wind and giving in to exhaustion. Breathing was an effort, and my leg muscles ached terribly." Then Maureen McGovern's pop song "Morning After" began to play over the loudspeakers, and he found himself swimming in time to the music. His tiredness vanished, and he felt as if he could swim forever. The next night, he experimented by swimming to the song again. His swimming was effortless. That particular song, Maharam concludes, "set a specific pace [that] got me to my peak."

Dr. Maharam has since studied endorphin levels in runners, using either naloxone or a saline placebo. He found that endorphins in the bloodstream did not necessarily correlate with mood or physical endurance. The runner's "high" may be more mysterious than we once thought. Though endorphins may be involved, other hormones and substances may trigger our feel-good mood.

One patient, a thirty-year-old advertising executive, goes to a special "spin" class at which participants ride lined-up exercise bikes while very intense popular music with a strong beat plays.

She described it this way:

Someone leads the class and tells you to step up, step down, go to the right, stand up on the bike, ride it standing, sit down on the bike, and move your shoulders from side to side, now we're going to pick up the pace with this song, now we're going to a slower song. I feel like I'm flying with it. It's like dance, there's something very pleasurable about moving your body to a specific rhythm. Exercising to music and rhythm is so powerful. After the class everyone feels wonderful, like they were high. We call it "spinner's high."

Whatever the cause of the exercise high, Maharam believes that each of us has a unique "golden mean," an optimum exercise level that is neither too minimal nor too exhausting. For more information about Maharam's exercise curve and how to use it, you may want to read his book.

WHAT IS FITNESS?

Fitness is made up of several factors: cardiorespiratory fitness (heart and lungs), muscular strength, and flexibility. Regular exercise will increase the amount of blood your heart can pump with each heartbeat. It will lower your heart rate when your body is at rest, improve your levels of cholesterol, lower your blood pressure, and reduce your body fat. Exercise will increase your energy, help you sleep better, and improve your mood.

Before you begin any kind of exercise program, it is important to check with your doctor, to be sure that you are not embarking on a routine that might aggravate a current health problem, such as arthritis or high blood pressure.

I've found that exercise programs succeed when they are both specific and fun. By specific, I mean setting attainable and concrete goals, such as increasing the number of sit-ups you do each day by five a week. By fun, I mean that you may include sports and activities like tennis and dancing, join a cycling club, go canoeing with friends, or engage in any number of activities that are exciting and entertaining. As Arnold Schwarzenegger has said, "People who turn fitness into a fun activity are the ones who end up doing it the rest of their lives."

HOW TO BEGIN

Sometimes it's hard to know just how and where to begin exercising. According to the American College of Sports Medicine, you can test your current fitness level. Their tests involve walking for a mile, doing push-ups and stretching and reaching exercises, and measuring yourself on charts to determine your fitness level. For more information, contact the American College of Sports Medicine at 317-637-9200.

EXERCISE: CAUSE AND CURE?

It's ironic, to say the least, that the most common asthma trigger besides allergy is exercise. About 80 percent of asthmatics and 40 percent of those with allergic rhinitis and hay fever suffer from exercise-induced asthma (EIA), according to Dr. Roger Katz of the University of California.

EIA may be caused by increased demand on twitchy airways, by breathing in polluted air, or perhaps by breathing rapidly through the mouth (so that air is not warmed and moistened by the nose). It is theorized that the loss of heat and water from the lungs results in a release of histamine, which may cause a spasm of the lungs. EIA can be triggered almost instantly—within a few minutes of beginning to exercise.

Yet exercise is also an effective way of managing asthma. Combined with proper breathing techniques, exercise can significantly improve aerobic function and lung capacity. It is estimated that up to 11 percent of elite athletes suffer from EIA. Tests of the 1984 U.S. Olympic team found that sixty-seven (11 percent) had EIA—yet they won forty-one medals. EIA does not necessarily mean you cannot exercise.

EIA symptoms usually begin within five minutes of starting to exercise and can include shortness of breath, wheezing, a sensation of tightness and burning in the chest, coughing, stomach pain, and fatigue. The sufferer may suddenly feel weak, and his or her performance or speed may plummet.

In some cases, EIA is the only form of asthma that an individual experiences and it may even go undiagnosed. The only obvious sign may be a cough after exercise, and yet in some cases lung capacity may be reduced as much as 85 percent. In particular, undiagnosed EIA in children can have severe consequences. Instead of complaining about their symptoms, they may simply withdraw from sports and athletics, without ever understanding why they are having trouble performing. In fact, according to the journal *Emergency Medicine*, any child who avoids exercise for no reason should be suspected of suffering from EIA.

Olympic swimmer Nancy Hogshead, author of *Asthma and Exercise*, explains that for an entire decade she swam competitively and never knew she had asthma. "I would sometimes feel unusually winded and tired during my workouts and competitions," she writes. "After some particularly hard training session or race, it wasn't uncommon for me to pass out momentarily at poolside."

At the Olympic Games in 1984, she swam the two-hundred-meter butterfly, the most grueling and demanding race of all, because of the difficulty and intensity of the stroke. "I found myself gasping for air in order to reach the end of the pool. . . . I got out of the pool coughing and wheezing." It was only then that an observant Olympic physician suggested she get tested for asthma.

Factors that can influence EIA include the following:

- Workouts in a cool, dry environment. Cold air can trigger EIA.
- Temperature. Autumn and early winter are times that many asthmatics suffer EIA attacks. The transition period from summer to autumn can also be particularly difficult.
- Breathing through the mouth while exercising. This does

not properly humidify and warm the air. In contrast, the mucous membranes of the nose swell slightly in the presence of cold air. This slows the passage of the air, allowing it time to be humidified and warmed.

- Allergies, including hay fever. During allergy season many asthmatics prefer to exercise indoors.
- Type of exercise. In general, vigorous cold-weather activities like skating, running, skiing, and sledding can cause a problem. Stop-and-go sports like football and baseball are far less likely to produce EIA, and tennis can often be tolerated by asthmatics. Swimming is recommended for most asthmatics because the air is warm and humid. However, a chemical- or mold-sensitive person may have trouble swimming in indoor pools. But keep in mind: EIA can occur at any time when a person is predisposed to it.

A NATURAL TREATMENT APPROACH TO EXERCISE AND ASTHMA

You may not realize how effective certain simple techniques can be in combating asthma, so that exercise is a pleasure. In particular, one form of training known as "pulsed" exercise can combat chronic illnesses like asthma at the same time it conditions the body.

Now that you have learned and are practicing your breathing techniques, you can apply them to any exercise program. In general, whenever you contract your body or part of your body, you should be breathing out and attempting to force out all the stale air in your lungs. Whenever you relax or expand your body, expand your lungs and breathe in. For instance, during a push-up, as you are lowering yourself to the floor and your hands are coming toward your body, you are contracting, so breathe out. Here's another example: during a sit-up or curl-up, you are contracting as you bring your chest into your knees, so breathe out. Then breathe in as you relax toward the floor.

You will find that in some cases, this is counter to your traditional experience of breathing. In weight lifting, for instance, you are told to breathe out when your hands are pushing the weights over your head, and to breathe in as your hands come down. But for an asthmatic, the opposite is recommended, at least with light weights. You are learning to take a deep breath against weight, against effort, against resistance, which allows you to bring air into all areas of your lungs and strengthens the chest muscles that you need during an asthma attack.

Before you begin any exercise program, you need to understand the importance of a warm-up period. EIA symptoms usually begin to flare within about five minutes of starting to exercise vigorously. If you start exercising slowly and extend your warm-up period, you can work through the asthma flare-up until the symptoms subside. Warm-up periods can last as long as half an hour. They work because they gradually prepare the lungs for the demands of exercise. Warm-up exercises can include stretching, slow calisthenics, and slow jogging and/or step routines. You can choose from the wide range of warm-up exercises recommended by qualified aerobics teachers or in fitness and exercise manuals.

If you wish to warm up with calisthenics and stretching exercises such as jumping, stretching, push-ups, and sit-ups, you may be interested to know that some routines are more effective than others. According to the American College of Sports Medicine, injury is more common with certain calisthenics. In addition, some exercises condition you better.

Specifically, the calisthenics that may cause injury include the following: Deep knee bends can be a strain for many individuals. Full sit-ups, with bent knees or straight legs, do not condition you as well as other types of sit-ups and may strain your back. Squat thrusts, donkey kicks, lying on your back and cycling your legs in the air, and double leg lifts can all cause muscle strain. Standing and touching your toes, circling your neck, or performing back bends are less effective than some other stretches.

More effective warmups include the following exercises:

1. Push-ups (wall push-ups)

With your palms flat against the wall at chest height, stand a few inches from the wall and push your body away from it. Or do push-ups with bent knees, keeping the body straight from knees to shoulders.

2. Curl-ups

Instead of sit-ups, do curl-ups. Bend your knees and slowly curl up until the middle of your back is off the floor. This is enough to develop your stomach muscles, and it will not strain your back. Doing curl-ups with straight legs does not work the stomach muscles, it works the hip flexor muscles. These muscles are often tight and need to be stretched, not strengthened.

You can do curl-ups with straight arms, arms crossed over your chest, or your hands on the floor.

3. Leg Lifts

To exercise your legs, you can lift them individually while lying on your stomach. You may lift the whole leg from the hip or bend the leg at the knee.

4. Leg Raises

To increase flexibility in your hips, you can lie on your side and slowly lift and lower your upper leg, keeping it straight. You can sit in a chair and raise your entire leg, keeping it straight. You can perform a stepping routine, stepping first with the right leg, then with the left.

5. Neck Stretch

You can simply turn your head slowly from side to side, as if you were looking both ways before crossing the street.

You can also do half-neck rolls: Slowly lower your head to the right, as if to lay your ear on your shoulder. Allow your head to slowly drop forward and roll to the left, until your left ear is above your shoulder. Then roll back to the right.

6. Shoulder Stretches

Raise your arms to the sky, stretching your sides. Do not bend your arms over your head. Circle your arms slowly from the shoulder, clockwise for several cycles, then counterclockwise for several cycles. Then roll your shoulders by rotating them while your hands are on your hips.

7. Leg Stretch

Lie on your back, and keep your knees slightly bent. Lift one leg, and grasp it at the slightly bent knee. Pull it toward your chest. Now bend your knee farther, and pull your leg in closer. Now do the same with the other leg.

8. Back Stretch

You can perform a modified version of the traditional yoga exercise known as the Cobra. Lie on the floor on your stomach, your forehead on the floor, and your arms bent with your palms flat on the floor on either side of your head. Lift your head and chest slowly, but keep your stomach on the floor.

9. Hip Stretches

Stand at a ninety-degree angle to the wall, with your hand lightly on the wall or the back of a chair for balance. Bend one leg at the knee and grasp your foot. Pull your foot toward your buttocks, stretching your leg and hip muscles. Change balancing hand and repeat with the other leg.

Sit on the floor, with the soles of your feet together and

your legs bent. Holding both feet with your hands, lean forward slowly as far as you can.

Sit on the floor with your legs straight. Now bend one leg at the knee, and place your foot on the outside of your other knee. Place your elbow on your upper thigh near your bent knee. Now twist your upper body away from your leg while you push against it with your elbow. Repeat on the other side.

During your warm-up, you may notice yourself sweating lightly. Breathe through your nose. Remember, the purpose of a warm-up period is to stretch, strengthen, and loosen your muscles, gradually increase your heart rate, and allow your lungs time to adapt to the increased demand for oxygen.

During the main period of vigorous exercise, try to breathe through your nose as much as you can. This can be difficult when you are really exercising hard, and you may find yourself breathing through your mouth at times. Don't panic. Just do the best you can.

In general, I recommend eight to twelve repetitions of most strengthening and flexing exercises.

PULSED EXERCISE

I find that brief, intense cycles of exercise and relaxation are often beneficial to asthmatics, whose lung capacity may not be great and who may be afraid to exercise for extended periods of time. I recommend a period of intense exercise of five minutes followed by two to three minutes of rest. However, I leave the cycles up to my patients or recommend using a peak flow meter. Check your peak flow numbers before exercising. After each exercise cycle, wait until your numbers return to normal, then resume. Or you can see what feels comfortable for you. Your pulse needs to drop by about 40 points, to within 10 points of your starting pulse.

Let's say my pulse was 80 when I began to exercise, and rose to 130 during my short cycle of intense activity. While I rest, I wait for it to drop to at least 90 before beginning to exercise again.

There is a device available called the Pulse Meter. It's a band that you put around your chest, along with a wrist-watch that transmits a signal to indicate exactly how fast your pulse is. It is available at many sporting goods stores. Otherwise you can take your pulse on your own, though it's a bit more difficult.

Pulsed exercise is easy to do with any type of exercise that you can easily start and stop. You can apply it to cycling, alternating brief periods of intense cycling and periods of coasting. You can apply it less easily with running, because most people who enjoy jogging seem to enjoy doing it steadily for several miles. But you can run a block, walk a block, run a block, and achieve a pulsed pattern this way.

Swimming is well-known for its emphasis on interval training, which includes short bursts of exercise. However, on first immersing yourself in water, it may feel cold, and constant movement may be required to keep your body temperature at a comfortable level. If that is a problem for you, starting and stopping may be a problem for you. Some of my patients enjoy pulsed swimming, and others do not.

Pulsed exercise can be easily applied to jumping rope, jumping on a trampoline, rowing machines, stair machines, and running machines. Some sports lend themselves to pulsed exercise. For instance, just taking a few moments to rest and do breathing exercises between points in a tennis match can be very helpful.

AEROBIC EXERCISE

Aerobic exercise can condition your lungs and offer you life-time benefits. Many asthmatics have poor aerobic capacity, which not only leads to problems with their illness but further damages their long-term health, increasing the risk of cardiovascular illness.

Any aerobic exercise demands that you attain a target heart rate for at least twenty minutes three times a week. To find your target rate, subtract your age from 220. Multiply the result by 65 percent and then by 85 percent. These are the low and the high range of your target heart rate.

Aerobic exercises include:

- Walking and race walking
- Jogging
- Swimming
- Cycling
- Cross-country skiing
- Rowing and canoeing
- Roller skating
- Climbing stairs
- Dancing
- Jumping rope, jumping jacks, step routines
- Aerobics classes
- Hiking and mountain climbing
- Tennis, racquetball, and squash

Aerobic activities such as running, jumping rope, and high-impact aerobics classes can be uncomfortable for some individuals. Low-impact aerobics such as swimming, cross-country skiing, and cycling are easier on the joints and just as effective.

Recent reports have shown that you can also condition yourself simply by increasing your daily activity. Walk for errands, take stairs instead of elevators, and generally try to be active as you go about your day. Walking is convenient and can be done anywhere in the world. "Walking is man's best medicine," claimed Hippocrates.

The following pointers will help you get the most from your aerobic exercise.

If you choose to race-walk, never allow both feet to leave the ground at the same time. One foot touches down before the other lifts up. Your legs do not bend at the knee nearly as much, and your movements are gliding. Arms are kept at a 90-degree angle and can swing from waist to chest.

If you choose to jog, you will burn up 35 more calories an hour than if you walk. To keep jogging fun, vary your routine. Take different routes, run with friends at times, or run to great music. There are adult running camps for joggers of any speed or skill.

If you choose to swim, keep in mind that your target heart rate will be about fifteen beats per minute slower than most other aerobic exercise. This is because the water cools your entire body and keeps your heart rate down. However, you will still burn calories as long as you swim vigorously. There is a common myth that swimmers do not lose weight as do other exercisers, but this is untrue unless you glide along slowly without effort. There are also programs available where one actually performs aerobic exercise, such as walking or jumping, in the pool without immersing your head in water.

One advantage of swimming is that it is unlikely to cause muscle injury. Another advantage is the humid air, which can be soothing to an asthmatic's lungs. On the other hand, swimming can be a problem for mold-sensitive asthmatics. Many indoor swimming pools are so humid they tend to grow mold along the tiles around the pool. In addition, heavy chlorine in some pools can be a problem for sensitive individuals. If your asthma seems to worsen after swimming, this exercise may not be a good choice for you.

Asthma can be worsened by excess weight. Exercise is an important part of my program for overweight asthmatics. Any serious program of weight loss should be supervised by your physician. If you are interested in losing weight, consider cross-country skiing or its equivalent, a skiing machine. This sport is a nearly perfect aerobic workout that tones the major muscle groups in your body. It also burns up more calories than other forms of exercise. Recent research found that exercises using a skiing machine burned over 1,000 calories an hour.

Remember, you can vary your exercise routine enormously. Consider these wild possibilities: For New Yorkers who like stair climbing, for instance, there is the annual "Empire State Run Up," sponsored by the New York Road Runners Club. Competitors run up 1,860 steps to the top of the Empire State Building. There is also a marathon in Colorado Springs where runners scale Pike's Peak, which is thirteen thousand feet high.

Seriously, now. For adults who want a trip down memory lane, back to their childhood days, jumping rope burns as many calories as jogging. Roller blading is one of the fastest growing sports in the country. And for the homebody, there is an endless stream of home video exercise programs.

PEAK PERFORMANCE: MIND AND BODY

Dr. Charles Garfield is a weightlifter who popularized a groundbreaking Eastern European discovery about the mind-body link in exercise. He found that by using mental preparation before bench pressing, he was able to lift much heavier weights much more rapidly than he had expected. Garfield used techniques like visualization, relaxation, and psyching himself up. When he began to utilize these techniques, he was pressing 280 pounds, and his goal was to reach 365 pounds within a year. After only an hour of mental preparation, he had reached his goal of 365 pounds!

Visualization is quite popular among both amateur and professional athletes. Before competing, they will visualize their successful performance in detail. They imagine the entire event, beginning with their warm-up, and see themselves as relaxed, powerful, smooth, and strong. Indeed, Elizabeth Manley, an Olympic figure skater, spent as much time on her mind as her body before the 1988 Olympics.

Visualization may work because, according to amazing recent research at Harvard University by Dr. Stephen Kosslyn, the mind responds to imagined images in the exact same way it responds to actual visual input. The same brain centers are stimulated, and the same memory circuits are activated.

As an asthmatic, you can visualize successful athletic performance along with easy breathing. In my own case, I have used visualization before beginning exercise. I imagine myself running a five-mile course, picturing the entire process and seeing myself breathing well. For instance, if I'm taking a run on the beach, I visualize certain landmarks and how good I'm going to feel as I run past them. This makes me feel psyched before I get started. In my mind, I have already seen myself successfully completing the activity. As I set out, I've already done it once and well in my head. The better I imagine it, and the greater the detail, the easier it is.

YOGA: AN ANCIENT AND PERFECT FORM OF EXERCISE

Yoga combines proper breathing with an exercise routine that strengthens muscles while ensuring flexibility. Certain forms of hatha or kundalini yoga offer substantial aerobic benefits and exercise the lungs well. It is almost a perfect form of fitness for the asthmatic. It can be very helpful because very few exercises emphasize the essential nature of breathing. In yoga, very specific belly breathing is required. I was recently on a talk show watching a yoga teacher perform her exercises, and I was astonished to find that deep breathing was required for every part of the exercise. It was a meditative and spiritual experience as well. See chapter 13 for a more detailed discussion.

WHAT ABOUT INHALERS?

Many asthmatics may wonder about the advisability of using an inhaler before exercise. The best approach is to determine your peak flow prior to exercise. In this way, you will know whether you are at risk for a problem during exercise. If your numbers are down 20 percent, you might indeed run into problems. If your numbers are good when you start to exercise, but you often experience asthma once you begin exercising, use Intal or Tilade. It is effective for EIA and can blunt the effects.

However, if your numbers are diminished, you may want to use Ventolin or an albuterol inhaler to get your numbers up to appropriate levels, and then perhaps take Intal as well. Take a puff, wait five minutes, check your peak flow numbers, and take another puff if necessary.

Of course, if you are involved in the CAP program in its entirety, over time you will need less and less medication. Your body will be stronger. I find that I turn to inhalers about 20 percent of the time during exercise. For instance, if I'm going to be involved in a very strenuous activity such as a very long run or a very competitive tennis match, I may take a puff or two before exercising. I find this far preferable to stopping during exercise and taking medication, when I do not exercise nearly as well.

In conclusion, exercise is an area that once was completely overlooked by many asthmatics, who were told to rest at home. Finding ways to help asthmatics exercise regularly is one of the most important things we can do to help them live long and well. The techniques discussed in this chapter can help asthmatics to attain proper aerobic tone and do so in a way that doesn't harm their system. The goal for a healthy person might be to run continuously for thirty minutes; for an asthmatic, it might be to run for a cumulative thirty minutes, even if it means stopping and starting in a pulsed fashion over the course of an hour.

We've learned that exercise is crucial for the health of virtually all asthmatics. It not only benefits our heart and lungs, it improves this chronic condition. No asthma program would be complete without a proper exercise routine.

DOCTOR'S RECOMMENDATIONS
FOR ACTION

1. Combine a breathing program with a regular exercise program. Aerobic fitness keeps the body oxygenated, improves lung function, and increases immunity. It also produces what is known as "runner's high," improving mood and well-being.

2. Check with your doctor before beginning any exercise program to be sure the routine is reasonable, given your state of health.

3. If you suffer from EIA, minimize it by avoiding workouts in a cool, dry environment; breathe through the nose to humidify the air; make sure the type of exercise you engage in is not aggravating your asthma (for instance, cold air may aggravate a skier's asthma, while the warm humid air of indoor swimming pools may be fine).

4. Make sure to engage in a warm-up period. If EIA symptoms flare, they usually do so within the first five minutes. Extend your warm-up period so that you can work through the asthma flare. Choose warm-ups such as wall and bent-knee push-ups, curl-ups instead of sit-ups, leg lifts and

leg raises, neck and shoulder stretches, and back and hip stretches.

5. If extended periods of exercise are difficult for you, try pulsed exercise.

6. Condition yourself by increasing daily activities. Walk to errands, take stairs instead of elevators, and generally try to be more active.

7. Practice visualization to increase aerobic fitness and strength. Visualize easy, open breathing and successful athletic performance before you begin to exercise.

8. Try yoga, a perfect form of exercise for asthmatics. It incorporates strengthening exercises with flexibility, stretching, and special breathing techniques.

9. Consider using an inhaler before exercise, but check your peak flow numbers first. If they are down 20 percent and you really want to work out, an inhaler may help. Intal is especially useful for EIA.

10. Start slowly. Have fun.

CHAPTER TWELVE

All in the Family

Childhood asthma affects approximately 10 million children in the United States. It causes more emergency room and hospital admissions and more missed school days than any other chronic illness of childhood. About a hundred thousand children in this country are hospitalized each year with bronchitis, and bronchitis often triggers asthma flare-ups. In fact, viral respiratory infection is the most common trigger of asthma attacks in children.

Half of all babies and young children wheeze from time to time, but as they grow, their airways also grow and often the wheezing stops. The children most likely to develop asthma are those whose airways are smaller than average. Children with normal-size airways who suffer from allergies and a family history of asthma will also be more likely to suffer from asthma.

Many a parent's worst nightmare is to see their child suffer from a chronic illness that makes it sometimes almost impossible to breathe. Almost inevitably, parents who bring their asthmatic children to me for treatment say they would gladly suffer all the wheezing, bronchitis, sleepless nights, and debilitation of this condition if only their child could be healthy.

The first thing I tell them is that, as debilitating as asthma can be for a child, it is in a sense the best time in life to have asthma. By adopting a program like CAP early in life, a child can avoid permanent lung damage, ensure that new lung tissue is healthy, and change the entire shape of his or her life. Even a child who has been frequently hospitalized or on high doses of medication can often become virtually symptom-free and healthy. Your child can swim, run, play baseball and basketball, perform well in school—just like any other child.

I feel that more and more physicians are coming to realize how important family involvement is in treating childhood asthma. Asthma is not just suffered by the patient. It is a family experience that affects mothers, fathers, siblings, and spouses, as well as close friends. Most important, each family's experience is distinct, as the following accounts demonstrate.

"Our son was hospitalized with asthma for the first time when he was only a year old," recalled Suzanne, a thirty-eight-year-old mother. "By the time he was three, he had been to the emergency room eight times. But that's not the worst of it. When he was four years old, he almost died of asthma. He caught a cold over the Christmas holidays, and of course, the doctor started him on antibiotics right away. But within two days, he was in the emergency room again. Except this time, both his lungs collapsed and he was put on a respirator for six days. The infection was so persistent he had to be put on intravenous antibiotics. It was a nightmare week. I practically lived, ate, and slept in the hospital. Miraculously, he recovered completely. But I can't say that I have. It's as if I can never get over it. I'm always scared of it happening again. He's eight years old now, but I worry every day and I know I'm overprotective of him, but I can't help it."

Asthma is a different experience for every family. In fact, for many families, it is the wear-and-tear of daily, chronic illness that is so difficult. While most people get bronchitis for a week and then bounce back to vitality and health, asthmatics suffer from chronic tightness, infections, and impairment of health.

"What is asthma to my daughter and me?" mused a twenty-nine-year-old father. "It's a grinding, tedious, day-after-day, drive-you-nuts illness that means she's never really well but never really ill. Sometimes she has a dry cough for weeks at a time. Not a terrible, hacking cough, but this little wheezing cough that just goes on all day long. You know the feeling you get when there's construction work outside your window, and you keep hearing the noise of jackhammers. Or how about Chinese water torture? I hear Cathy's cough and there's nothing I can do and I feel terrible. She can't run and play like other kids because she gets attacks from exercise, especially in the winter. She wakes up at night wheezing. But when my wife and I used to take Cathy to our pediatrician, he'd tell us we were lucky that her asthma was under control and she'd never been hospitalized. Finally I decided that even though her illness was not life threatening, it was taking too much of life away from her. That's why we started on the CAP program. Our story, anyway, has a fairy-tale ending. With this program, she's become virtually asymptomatic. It wasn't an easy haul, changing her diet, stripping the house of carpet, taking away her stuffed animals, and teaching her breathing exercises every day. But it was worth it!"

"I think the hardest part about Mark's asthma for me was that during the day he looked healthy, and other parents would say to me, 'But he looks fine. He looks normal,' " said another patient of mine. "It was at night when I'd be awakened to face the total panic of a child who couldn't breathe. I'd give him medicine in a nebulizer or run the shower in the bathroom until it was filled with steam, and sit with him there for half an hour or an hour. Finally, he'd be okay and I'd put him to bed and it was me who'd lie awake for another hour, going to his room every fifteen minutes to make sure he was okay. But other parents don't know about that. And they don't know how hard our whole family worked to help Mark. We gave away our beautiful German shepherd, ran top-of-the-line air filters in the furnace and his bedroom, changed his sheets every other day, sprayed his bedding to reduce dust mites, watched his diet, and checked his peak flow meter every morning and evening. His health improved, but even so, more than once a well-meaning friend would imply that somehow we were to blame for Mark's bronchitis in the winter or allergic asthma during hay fever season."

When treating asthmatic children, I try to keep in mind that in a sense a whole family is suffering from this condition. The entire family, therefore, needs to understand the CAP program. A child of any age can go through most steps of CAP with help from a concerned and supervising parent and physician. (You can even check babies for allergies through blood tests.) All that this book has taught you about a complete asthma protocol—from dietary changes to supplements, breathing, environmental cleanup, and the whole panoply of techniques that make up CAP—are applicable to children. The difference is that when a child has asthma, the parents need to be closely involved in preventing and treating attacks.

I have many specific hints that I teach parents to help their asthmatic children. I emphasize education, prevention, and involvement. But most of all I emphasize structure. The parents of my pediatric patients are often extremely busy. Many have two-career households and other children. It is important for these parents to know as much as possible about their child's asthma.

I teach parents to handle many problems at home without an office visit, how to judge the severity of each symptom, and how to use a peak flow meter, stethoscope, and nebulizer. Just as important, I stress clearly demarcated goals and rules. Children need structure. They respond well to tools like charts with stars or blocks of color for taking medication on time, as well as rewards (from a good video to a tasty treat) for following the CAP program successfully.

AT THE DOCTOR'S OFFICE: YOUR CHILD AND YOU

One of the most significant functions a doctor can perform for a family in which one or more members suffer from asthma is to *listen* to them. As more than one parent has complained, "I'm the one who lives with my child. I know when something is wrong. Why do some doctors assume they can treat my child without involving me? I want to learn to help. And they should know that sometimes I'm just as scared as my child, but I'm the one who *has* to remain calm. I need help, too."

Help comes in the form of education and specific guidelines for treatment that the whole family can work on. I suggest to parents that before they visit their physician, they write down their questions and concerns. I also recommend that during the office visit, they take notes about symptoms, the results of any lab or allergy tests, and the doctor's impressions and instructions.

You can do a lot to help your child's health by keeping a daily symptom diary. List symptoms like cough, wheezing, runny or clogged nose, sleep problems, shortness of breath, fatigue, or pallor. Notice if the chest skin seems sucked in when your child tries to breathe in. Look especially at the skin between the ribs and above the collarbone. Try to observe if your child takes longer to breathe out, since during asthma attacks breathing out can take twice as long as breathing in. Is your child breathing faster?

Normal breathing rates per minute are as follows: 25 to 60 for infants, 20 to 30 for children under four years, 15 to

25 for children five to eighteen. When a child is sleeping, breathing is normally slower. Sometimes during an asthma attack, your child will be wheezing so loudly you can hear it across the room. Your child may also complain that his neck feels funny. He may scratch under his chin or at his throat, complaining that it itches.

In many children, a cough is the first sign of an asthma flare-up. An asthmatic cough is usually high, short, and frequent. In some children, a cough is the only obvious sign of underlying asthma.

For your child, especially a young child, visits to the doctor may be feared or resented. This is often the case for toddlers who are afraid of needles and allergy testing. More than once a terrified child has wept and wailed in holy terror just at the sight of a needle for drawing blood.

Before a visit to the doctor, you may want to explain to your child just what is going to happen. Tell her that the doctor may put some special medicine on her arm or back (scratch or prick tests), and it may hurt for a moment, but it will help the doctor figure out how she can get well. Let her know that you will hold her and she can cry if she wants, but that she must keep still so the medicine can work.

Bring along some favorite treats or a favorite stuffed animal or a new toy for her to unwrap after her "ordeal." Give the toy if your child has behaved well at the office. You can also create a kind of game by putting stickers or stars in a special notebook or a chart on the bedroom wall in reward for good behavior. A certain number of stickers or stars can be cashed in for a present.

MEDICAL CARE AT HOME:
WHAT YOU CAN DO

You can learn to perform certain procedures at home that can greatly reduce doctor's visits and help you and your child manage his or her asthma efficiently.

First, use a peak flow meter regularly. As I have discussed elsewhere, the peak flow meter is a handheld instrument that has been in use for over two decades. Like a thermometer, which measures body temperature, a peak flow meter measures air pressure. The patient simply takes a deep breath and blows as hard as possible into the meter. The force of the breath moves an arrow along the metered cylinder. This procedure is repeated a few times, and the highest number is recorded and compared to the normal range, which can be established in the physician's office or by using the peak flow meter when your child feels perfectly fine. A child whose peak flow rate is 75 percent of his or her personal best may have no symptoms while resting, but if exercising or exposed to allergens, symptoms will flare.

Peak flow meters provide important and accurate information about just how tight the lungs are. Children will often insist they are fine even when they are wheezing. They may argue and refuse to take their medicine. By using the peak flow meter, parent and child can determine just what is really happening. Peak flow meters can also help give a child confidence: if the reading is normal, the child will often feel more comfortable about playing with friends. Most children age four and above can comfortably blow into a peak flow meter.

The peak flow rate varies over a twenty-four-hour time period. It is usually lowest between midnight and morning.

See *Resources* on page 305 for information about obtaining a good peak flow meter.

Also check your child's breathing with a stethoscope.

Your doctor can teach you how to listen to each of the sections, or quadrants, of the lungs as your child inhales and exhales. The pitch and loudness of "windy" noises indicates the severity of an attack. If you hear high-pitched sounds only at the end of an exhalation, the attack is mild or just beginning. If you hear the sounds for the entire exhalation, the attack is more severe.

The stethoscope can be invaluable for toddlers who cannot express in words that they are wheezing and cannot describe how they feel.

After checking breathing with a peak flow meter and stethoscope, you can phone the doctor and give him the information. The doctor will be able to accurately prescribe medication in many cases. These two instruments are invaluable for nighttime asthma as well. Many parents find that their children suffer attacks during the night, but at the doctor's office in the bright light of day, they seem fine. A parent can feel frustrated by the situation and may be afraid of being labeled overprotective or paranoid by the physician. I've known a parent or two who withheld medication from an asthmatic child during the night, not out of maliciousness, but in order to "prove" the child was ill the next day at the doctor's.

By monitoring a child's breathing during the night with these instruments and recording the results, every parent has an accurate report of just what happened during the night. For example, "At 11 P.M. John woke up coughing and wheezing. His peak flow reading was x. There was a high-pitched whining sound upon exhalation in the right quadrant of his lungs. At 2 A.M. he woke again with an attack. His peak flow reading was y."

Home use of a nebulizer can reduce visits to the doctor and prevent emergency room admissions. Nebulizers are portable air compressors that transform liquid into a mist. The mist is inhaled by the patient. Many bronchodilators, such as Alupent and Ventolin, are used in nebulizers, as is

Intal. Nebulizers can be a great boon to children and even to infants. They deliver asthma medication very effectively and are especially helpful when lung function is impaired.

Spacers can help children to direct the spray of an inhaler properly. A spacer is a tube that fits onto the mouthpiece of an inhaler, directing the spray into the patient's mouth more easily. This increases the amount of medication that makes it into the airways. For infants, a mask with a breathe valve on it, which lets you know when your baby has breathed the medicine in, is available. Though infants may not like the device, it can be helpful.

For sinus trouble, Water Pik makes a nasal attachment that can be used with aloe vera juice and salt, the formula described earlier, to create a soothing, antiinflammatory and antibacterial solution that can help clear out the sinuses. If this is done on a regular basis, it can help your child avoid the head colds and sinus infections that sometimes lead to an acute attack of bronchitis.

HELPING YOUR CHILD
TAKE MEDICINE PROPERLY

Here are a few tips for parents:
- Make sure to use a proper measuring spoon, not a soup or dinner spoon from your set of silver. It's important that amounts of medication be exact, especially since many asthma medications contain strong substances like cortisone.
- For infants, purchase a liquid-medicine dispenser at the drugstore. It looks like a big fat plastic eyedropper. Fill the dispenser to the appropriate level and squirt the medication on the back of your baby's tongue or toward the inside cheek.
- If your baby spits up the medicine, buy a dispenser that has a nipple at the top. The baby will automatically suck before it tastes the medicine.

- If necessary, hold your infant's nose until he opens his mouth, and then squirt in the medicine.
- If children have trouble swallowing capsules, open them and sprinkle them on treats like pudding or sweetened yogurt.
- Help your child get into the habit of taking medicine regularly by rewarding her for it. You can make a chart, hang it on the wall, and have your child put a star on the chart each time she takes prescribed medicine. At the end of the week, add up the stars and give your child a treat such as a favorite video, food, or activity.

A SAFE HAVEN: YOUR CHILD'S BEDROOM

As I have already made clear in this book, environmental toxins and allergens can be powerful triggers of asthma. In fact, studies have shown that the level of dust mites in a home is linked to early onset of wheezing. Consider the fact that children also play on floors polished and cleaned with chemicals, or on synthetic carpets that may be outgassing toxins. Also, your home may contain molds, perfumes, cigarette smoke, and many other irritants. It is crucial, then, that your child's bedroom, where he or she plays and sleeps, be a safe haven.

I suggest the following steps to parents of asthmatic children:

1. Reduce bedroom dust. Buy vinyl or cotton-polyester casings to protect mattresses and pillows from dust mites. You may want to encase boxsprings as well. If your doctor prescribes these, they can be a tax-deductible medical expense.

2. Wash all bedding weekly to kill any new dust mites.

3. Keep books, toys, and other dust-collecting items to a minimum. You may have to tell your child that his or her

beloved stuffed animals need to sleep in another room, or store them in a clear plastic toy box with a lid, or in a bookcase. Buy vinyl or plastic animals (children love the Stretch-Man, for instance) as a substitute.

4. Vacuum carpets weekly. Shampoo them monthly. Better yet, remove carpeting from your child's bedroom. Wipe woodwork, closets, and drawers every few days with a damp rag. Replace heavy drapery or venetian blinds with washable curtains or shades.

5. Keep humidity in your child's room between 25 and 40 percent if you can. Air that is too dry can be uncomfortable, but humidity over 40 percent can stimulate the growth of molds and mites.

6. Replace any standard filters in a forced-air heating system with electrostatic air precipitators, which will filter and clean the air. You can buy these filters from air-conditioning distributors. Have the air ducts in your home cleaned. Our heating and cooling systems often contain contaminants and molds such as aspergillus and penicillium. You can check air ducts with a flashlight by removing the vent covers and looking inside. Clean air ducts improve fuel efficiency.

7. Purchase a HEPA air filter for your child's bedroom. Austin Air makes one of the best filters on the market.

8. Purchase a high-quality vacuum made for people with allergies. Some models include Nilfisk, Vita-Vac, and Euroclean. Unlike regular vacuums, which often stir up dust, these models are exceptionally effective at collecting it. You can also buy a specially designed filter for regular vacuums. These filters are made for trapping allergens.

SHARING FEELINGS

One aspect of a chronic illness like asthma is that it gives rise to emotions and worries in both parents and children. Often these emotions are kept hidden, but they take their toll on physical and mental health. I encourage parents to talk to me and to other parents of asthmatic children, so that they will learn many of their feelings and worries are normal. Here are some common feelings:

- My child is different from other children.
- My child is frustrated he cannot do everything other children do.
- My child is anxious, afraid, and cautious.
- I'm being overprotective, but I can't help myself.
- I'm not certain I'm doing the right thing for my child.
- I wish I could breathe for my child.
- I'm upset because I miss so many nights of sleep as a result of my child's asthma.
- I cannot help my child enough because she ignores asthma until the attack is severe.
- It's hard to get my child to take his medication on time.
- My child "uses" asthma to get attention.
- My spouse is angry because I spend too much time with my asthmatic child.
- I'm worried about the long-term effects of medication.
- I feel guilty because asthma comes from my side of the family.
- I'm angry at my spouse because asthma runs on his side of the family.

All the above feelings are quite common, and parents are often relieved to find their response to caring for an asthmatic child is shared by others.

THE BIG DRAMA: FAMILY PETS

Saying good-bye to the family pet can be a difficult ordeal, especially if one child in the family has asthma and others do not. There may be weeping, accusations, fights, and a period of mourning. Even though, in the abstract, the choice between a child and a pet seems clear, it can be incredibly hard to let go of a beloved pet. More than one parent has found a family pet a new home, only to hear this from the new owners: "Spot is dying of a broken heart. He won't eat. He hides under the couch. Maybe if he had a visit from you."

Some families will try to compromise by keeping a pet in a certain part of the house. Even so, an allergic or asthmatic child will often disobey the rules and play with the pet or invite it to sleep in the bedroom. If a child with asthma is allergic to a pet, keeping one in the house is like actively harming that child's health.

I suggest the following considerations to families with pets:

- Realize that cats and dogs with short hair can cause just as many allergies as long-haired animals. Short hair is not a solution for an asthmatic or allergic child.
- Understand that the real cause of pet allergies are the proteins found in saliva and urine, which are often carried on animal fur.
- If you are uncertain just how much of a problem your pet might be for your child, but your child seems to be suffering and their asthma has worsened since acquiring the pet, ask your doctor to test your child for allergy to your pet. Find a temporary home for the pet for at least two months, completely clean and vacuum the house and air it out, and see if your child's allergies improve. Remember, children may love their pet but it's important for you to put their health first.
- Try keeping pets like tropical fish, frogs, snails, turtles, birds, and so forth. However, all pets must be kept clean. Or, in warmer climates, you may be able to keep your pet outside and build them a special place to sleep.

ASTHMA AND SCHOOL

Even if you work as hard as possible to clean up your home, your child will still be attending school every day. Schools can be notorious hot spots for asthmatic or allergic children. Dust from chalk and blackboards, chemicals used to clean floors and walls, windows kept shut during the winter, inadequate ventilation, heating and cooling systems that haven't been properly cleaned in years—all these can lead to a school environment that is difficult for a child. Even waiting on the corner for the school bus every day can be a problem, if the bus belches out exhaust as it pulls up.

Make an effort to protect your child by talking to the teacher and the principal. Let them know your asthma protocol and how they might help your child. Give specific instructions about calling you if certain signs of an attack are present. Leave an inhaler or other emergency medication with the teacher after showing him or her how to use it. You may even want to instruct the teacher on using a peak flow meter. Let the school personnel know that chalk dust, plants, pollens, and chemicals used in science projects or in cleaning can all trigger asthmatic episodes. If there is a school nurse, be sure to talk with him or her. Also let the gym or physical education teacher know if there are any limitations on your child's ability to engage in sports and exercise. Dusty gyms can be a problem for asthmatic children.

The key to successful treatment of a pediatric patient is education. The doctor must educate the parents, who must in turn educate their child and other important figures in the child's life—from teachers to friends to relatives. Remember, the early years of an asthmatic's life are critical times. Asthma in childhood is both a crisis and an opportunity. With proper treatment, most asthmatic children can become truly active and vital—ensuring that their natural birthright of health is restored and preserved.

RESOURCES

Peak flow meters are available from many manufacturers. Most companies make a low-flow-range model for children under the age of five, and a full-range model for adults. Good peak flow meters should last several years and should be easy to hold and to read. The National Heart, Lung, and Blood Institute (301-251-1222, P.O. Box 30105, Bethesda, MD 20824-0105) has established guidelines for peak flow meters. For more information, look for *A User's Guide to Peak Flow Monitoring,* by Dr. Guillermo Mendoza and Debbie Scherer.

Several types of nebulizers are available. The standard consists of a motor with a filter, masking, and tubing. Some models offer nasal tips, batteries, or adapters for car cigarette lighters. For young children, a home nebulizer that allows the patient to lie down while breathing is advised. For children who like to camp or play sports, a portable, battery-operated unit is often worth the extra cost. New nebulizers can cost from $125 to $400; reconditioned units can sometimes be found for as little as $25. You will also need to purchase replacement cups, tubing, and filters. Most nebulizer cups can be used several times if properly cleaned; some are part of the machine itself and are never replaced.

The following organizations can provide useful materials and products for asthma sufferers and their families:

- American Lung Association, 1740 Broadway, NY 10019, 800-LUNG-USA, provides information on asthma camps, asthma school programs, research grants.
- Asthma and Allergy Foundation of America, 1125 15th

Street, N.W., Suite 502, Washington, DC 20005, 202-466-7643, Ext. 226 for publications.

- Center Laboratories, 35 Channel Drive, Port Washington, NY 11050, 800-2-CENTER, peak flow meters, spacers, EpiPen, Multi-Test allergy kits.
- Clement Clarke, Inc., 3128 East 17th Ave., Suite D, Columbus, OH 43219, 800-848-8923, offers peak flow meters and sonic mist nebulizers.
- Klaire Laboratories, Inc., 1573 West Seminole, San Marcos, CA 92069, 800-533-7255, aloe vera juice, supplements, etc.
- N.E.E.D.S. (National Ecological and Environmental Delivery System), 527 Charles Ave., Suite 12A, Syracuse, NY 13209, 800-711-1123, offers a catalogue of products for allergic and asthmatic persons.
- Nilfisk of America, 300 Technology Drive, Malvern, PA 19355, 800-NILFISK, manufactures vacuums and peak flow meters.
- Sedna Specialty Health Products, P.O. Box 1453, Andrews, NC 28901, 800-223-0858, offers products for allergic individuals and special asthma formulas for children.

DOCTOR'S RECOMMENDATIONS FOR ACTION

1. If your child has asthma, recognize that by taking the initiative to treat him or her now with a program like CAP, you can prevent any long-term damage.

2. Family involvement is crucial in treating childhood asthma. The entire family needs to understand how to manage asthma and how to utilize the CAP program.

3. Know that many asthmatic flare-ups can be handled at home and may require only a phone call to the doctor if you are a properly informed parent:

- Learn how to use a nebulizer, a peak flow meter, and a stethoscope. By using a peak flow meter, you will have an objective tool to determine if your child needs medication.
- Ask your doctor to work with you so that he can prescribe proper medication over the phone when necessary.
- Use a nebulizer at home to reduce emergency visits to the doctor or hospital.
- Use spacers to help children direct inhaler sprays.
- Give children tools like charts with stars or blocks of color for taking medication on time, as well as rewards.
- Keep a daily symptom diary for your child. Note symptoms like cough, wheezing, sleep problems, fatigue, and pallor.
- Know what normal breathing rates are for your child's age.
- Let your child know just what will happen at a visit to the doctor's, and bring along favorite treats as rewards for good behavior in young children.
- Make sure your child's bedroom is a safe haven free of allergens, dust, and toxins.
- Give your child time to share feelings about asthma, and make sure you have a place to discuss your own feelings.
- If your child suffers from allergies to pets, try to keep non-allergenic pets like fish, turtles, and birds.
- Talk to the teacher and principal at your child's school. Let them know about your asthma protocol and how they might help your child. Let them know the warning signs of an attack. Leave emergency medicine with your child's teacher after instructing him or her how to use it.

CHAPTER THIRTEEN

Mind and Body: Effective Healing Techniques

Throughout history there have been stories of miraculous cures, spontaneous remissions, mysterious healings. One of my favorite stories is that of a man known in the medical literature simply as "Mr. Wright," who twice escaped the jaws of death merely because of so-called false hope.

Mr. Wright was dying of cancer of the lymph nodes, and according to his physician, Dr. Philip West, had huge tumor masses the size of oranges. His doctors expected him to die within a few weeks, but when Mr. Wright heard that a new drug called Krebiozen was going to be tested, he begged to be included in the study. He was so ill he couldn't get out of bed. His first injection was given on a Friday; on the following Monday, walking and chatting happily, he came to the clinic. "The tumor masses melted like snowballs on a hot stove," reported the astonished doctor, "and in only these few days, they were half their original size!" Within ten days he was nearly well.

The miracle might have ended there, except that within a few months the study results revealed that the drug was useless. Mr. Wright "began to lose faith in his last hope . . . and after two months of practically perfect health,

he relapsed to his original state." The doctor, aware now of
the power of his patient's faith, decided to tell Mr. Wright
the drug *was* effective after all and that a new, double-
strength dose would now be given.

The doctor reports: "Mr. Wright, as ill as he was, became
his optimistic self again. . . . With much fanfare, I administered the first injection—consisting of fresh water and nothing more. Recovery from his second near-terminal state was
even more dramatic. Tumor masses melted, chest fluid vanished. . . . The water injections were continued, since they
worked such wonders. He then remained symptom-free for
over two months."

But once again, the miracle did not hold. The final
announcement from the American Medical Association
appeared in the press: "Nationwide tests show Krebiozen to
be a worthless drug in treatment of cancer."

Mr. Wright died a few days later.

You don't have to believe in psychic forces to be fascinat-
ed by the mind's power to heal and by the remarkable effect
of techniques that help bring the mind and body into
harmony. The body, after all, is its own pharmacy, manufac-
turing powerful "drugs" such as cortisone, opiate-like
chemicals, adrenaline, and the myriad neurotransmitters
that psychotropic medications like Prozac address.
Although this chapter speaks of mind *and* body, it is probably more correct to view them as one thing—the "mind-
body" that is each individual.

From biofeedback to meditation, yoga to self-hypnosis,
visualization to tai chi, there are outstanding approaches
that can help you reset and regulate the immune system. I
recommend to all my patients that they sample the wide
range of mind-body healing methods available, several of
which I describe in this chapter, and I consider this part of
the CAP program as important as aerobic exercise and
breathing properly.

Each patient will have his or her own preference. I prefer meditation and visualization; some of my patients are devotees of yoga (which many studies have shown to be particularly effective for asthma); still others find biofeedback to be extremely helpful. The choice, of course, is yours.

One patient of mine, Bob, is a thirty-nine-year-old life insurance executive who has had asthma since childhood. His drug diet consisted of beta-agonist sprays, theophylline, and occasional cortisone. He complained of feeling constantly jittery and nervous, and so as part of his CAP protocol I gave him three training sessions in meditation, visualization, and self-hypnosis.

The first week I taught him a simple method of meditation. The second week, after he had relaxed into a meditative state, I asked him to visualize a beach with crystal-clear deep blue skies and crystalline waters lapping against the beach. Then I asked him to imagine himself in a sailboat, blowing the sails so the boat sped along gaily, then resting so the boat skimmed slowly, then blowing the sails again. In his third session, we added a self-hypnosis technique called autosuggestion. He chose a key word, placed his hand over his sternum, and was instructed to feel heat in his hand and then to sense that warming heat filling and relaxing his lungs. Whenever he needed to feel that warmth and relaxation in the future, he was to place his hand over his sternum and say that key word.

Once these techniques become familiar, the body becomes conditioned to respond to them quickly. That conditioned response (warmth, relaxation, opening of the lungs) can be achieved rapidly, and many individuals become so adept at the techniques they can use them anytime and anyplace.

"I use the techniques you taught me four or five times a day," Bob says. "They are just invaluable. They have allowed me to cut my sprays down by half. I don't know how it can work so well, but it sure does!"

How does the mind-body connection work? According to Dr. J. Allan Hobson, a professor of psychiatry at Harvard Medical School and a member of the MacArthur Foundation Mind-Body Network, "The brain-mind has its own built-in healing power. Unfortunately, until you have a grasp of how it heals itself, you are as likely to interfere with the process as you are to help it. You can improve your health—both mental and physical—by voluntarily changing states." And you can do that through the techniques surveyed in this chapter.

For those of you who might be a bit skeptical, scientific research has actually shown how a person's belief in a treatment might influence the healing process. Nearly twenty years ago, groundbreaking laboratory experiments found that the immune system could be conditioned, in just the same way that Ivan Pavlov conditioned dogs to salivate at the ringing of a bell. Two researchers, psychologist Robert Ader and immunologist Nicholas Cohen at Rockefeller University gave rats a taste of saccharin water and followed it with an injection of a drug that causes temporary sickness and suppresses the immune system. The rats learned to associate the taste of saccharin with the drug's effects. Later, when they were given saccharin water followed by a harmless injection of saltwater, they reacted just as if they had been given the drug: they got sick and their immune systems were suppressed.

The mind has power to heal the body and boost immune response as well. At the National Institutes of Health, Novera Herbert Spector exposed mice to the harmless odor of camphor at the same time that he injected them with an immune-boosting drug. After nine rounds of this treatment, just a sniff of camphor alone increased the potency of the rats' natural killer cells.

These studies confirm what science has long known simply through experience. For instance, a 1959 analysis of fifteen double-blind studies found that 35 percent of patients with a wide variety of postoperative pain obtained relief with placebos (inert sugar pills). A later 1985 review of eleven more double-blind studies found that 36 percent of patients experienced a 50 percent reduction in pain when taking placebos. (Double-blind means that neither the patients nor the doctors knew who was receiving actual pain medication and who was receiving a harmless placebo.) In fact, a wide range of studies have found that the placebo effect can provide significant and even therapeutic relief in a variety of conditions, including hypertension, diabetes, ulcers, asthma, arthritis, and other illnesses.

Simply making an appointment to see a doctor may have a significant placebo effect. In one much discussed proof of the power of placebo, an anti-ulcer drug was tested in the United States and England before it was approved. Seventy percent of patients on placebo and 80 percent on the drug were healed of their ulcers in England. In America, 80 percent of patients on placebo and 90 percent on the drug were healed. Those extraordinarily high numbers indicate the power of placebo in stress-related illness.

Researchers wanted to know why there was a 10 percent difference between England and America. When they examined the study protocol, they found that in England, patients were sent their medication with instructions in the mail, while in America doctors administered the medication. It seems that the mere contact with a doctor was enough to hike up the placebo cure another 10 percent, so that an astounding eight out of ten patients were cured simply through the power of the mind.

In one fascinating experiment conducted in 1958, placebo surgery was performed on randomly selected patients. The skin was simply opened and closed, and patient recovery was compared to those who had received an operation. Patients treated with a placebo operation remained improved for at least six months.

Just how does the mind influence the body? It turns out that the brain and the immune system speak the same chemical language. Nerve cells in the brain send signals to each other with proteins called polypeptides. White blood cells produce the same polypeptides, which signal the immune system to produce antibodies and other chemicals that fight infection. Both the brain and the immune system can respond to the other's chemical signals. In fact, white blood cells have receptors for hormones and neurotransmitters. Lymph tissue (in the bone marrow, thymus, spleen, tonsils, and lymph nodes) is filled with nerves, and cells deep in the brain have receptors for the chemicals the immune system produces.

That means that the brain and immune system form a continuous feedback loop, influencing and being influenced by the other.

Scientists speculate that the immune system is a kind of sixth sensory system, one that recognizes the substances we can't see or touch (such as viruses). The immune system then produces specific hormones to signal the brain about what is happening in the body.

In fact, some scientists believe both the brain and immune system developed from the same ancestral cells. Both systems can learn and remember. As Dr. Lewis Thomas has written, the two master systems join together to form "a kind of superintelligence that exists in each of us."

Let's examine just how we can access that superintelligence and help it to help us. Perhaps the key to the effectiveness of most mind-body techniques is the ability to relax. Relaxation has profound beneficial effects on immunity and health.

Studies of a specific class of the body's white blood cells—neutrophils—have found that they function significantly better when individuals are trained to relax. (Neutrophils are the samurai warriors of the blood and are crucial in protecting us against bacteria and viruses.) When students were trained over six sessions to relax and visualize improving the function of their neutrophils, they were able to greatly increase or decrease the number of neutrophils circulating in the blood. This was merely through the influence of the mind. Not a single drug was used. An important point here is that the students could modulate their immune system in either direction. This is significant in any inflammatory condition, including asthma, for inflamed tissue attracts neutrophils and leads to further inflammation. Imagery and visualization can actually heal inflamed tissue.

As you read the rest of this chapter, keep in mind that in many ways it is a companion piece to the chapter on the importance of breath. Virtually all the mind-body techniques that follow benefit from deep, abdominal breathing.

MEDITATION

In many different countries, across recorded time, man has meditated in an attempt not only to find peace and relaxation but to expand awareness and reach a fuller state of being. From India to Syria, Japan to China, medieval European monasteries to modern Zen retreats, meditation has been a common practice. Meditation connects us with what George Leonard in *The End of Sex* calls "the heart of each of us, whatever our imperfections, [where] there exists a silent pulse of perfect rhythm—a complex of wave forms and resonances which is absolutely individual and unique and yet which connects us to everything in the universe." And according to Chogyam Trungpa Rinpoche, one of the most widely followed Tibetan teachers in the world, in *Cutting Through Spiritual Materialism*, "When performing the meditation practice, one should develop the feeling of opening oneself out completely to the whole universe with absolute simplicity and nakedness of mind."

Experienced practitioners of meditation sometimes compare the training and tuning of the mind to an athlete's disciplined training of his body. Studies have shown that meditation produces a physiological state of profound relaxation, while the mind is still awake and alert. The metabolism slows down, as does the heart and breath. The blood lactate level (an indication of anxiety and tension) drops sharply during meditation. Brain waves in the alpha level, which is associated with relaxation, increase. The resistance of skin to mild electric current rises by as much as 400 percent, indicating a state of profound calm. (Skin resistance decreases as inner anxiety and tension increase.)

In 1968, Dr. Herbert Benson and colleagues at Harvard Medical School tested volunteer practitioners of Transcendental Meditation to see if it could really counter stress. Their scientific measurements proved that heart and breathing really did slow down, oxygen consumption fell by 20 percent, blood lactate levels really did drop, skin resistance did increase fourfold, and brain-wave patterns showed an increase in alpha waves. Benson also went on to show, in further studies, that any typical meditation practice could produce these physiological changes. Since that time meditation has been used to help treat high blood pressure, heart disease, stroke, migraine headaches, and even autoimmune diseases such as arthritis. It is definitely a useful method for asthma.

Meditating can be difficult because it is hard to be still and focused. Each time your mind wanders, simply bring it gently back to the object of your focused attention, whether it is your breath, a word, a phrase, a candle flame, or simply the vast pool of being. Patients sometimes come to me and say, "I can't do it. My mind won't stay still." I tell them it may take weeks or months before they can train their mind to be still, and even if the mind wanders, that's okay.

When you meditate, you can sit in a comfortable chair with your hands resting in your lap, sit cross-legged on the floor with a cushion under your buttocks, in a full lotus position (as taught in yoga), or you can even do it lying down. Don't worry about the amount of time you spend meditating—you can begin with just a few minutes a day and eventually build up to twenty minutes twice a day.

There are different forms of meditation: **One-pointed meditation** requires that you look at an object and simply concentrate on it. Give it all your attention. You will notice that, again and again, your mind will drift away and you will start thinking of something else. Bring your attention back to the object. You may feel sleepy or irritable or want to keep moving and shifting because of sudden aches, pains, or itches. Or you may find that the object itself seems to take on almost supernatural colors or auras or to shift in size. That is due to your mind's restlessness and need for stimulation. Rather than let yourself be distracted, simply continue to observe.

You can choose any object for one-pointed meditation. Many people like to use a candle flame. It has enough inherent variety to capture your attention.

Breath counting is a form of meditation that is just what it says: one simply counts the breath. It is common in Zen buddhism, where one counts ten breaths in a row, and then begins again. You may want to count to three or four, or you could count this way: one (inhale) and two (exhale) and three (inhale) . . . and so on. Choose whichever way of counting is comfortable for you. Try to incorporate this in a session that includes the breathing exercises in this book.

You can meditate by **chanting** a word again and again. This is often called "mantra meditation." Some common chants are "Om," "Om shanti," "Om namah shivaya," "God is one," "All is peace," "Choose joy." You can chant your mantra silently to yourself or aloud. Try to be aware of each syllable as you pronounce it.

You can perform **open-focus meditation, or mindfulness**. Mindfulness involves simply being aware, witnessing

all of life without judgment. Begin by becoming a specta-
tor of your own stream of consciousness, your own emotions,
your own physical sensations. Don't try to stop them or
change them, just let them be. Observe. You will quickly
learn that the part of you that is observing the "rest" of you
is a separate part. That part can always be peaceful.

Here is a mindfulness meditation, created by Zen master
Thich Nhat Hanh:

Breathing in, I know I am breathing in.

Breathing out, I know I am breathing out.

Breathing in, I see myself as a flower.

Breathing out, I feel fresh.

Breathing in, I see myself as a mountain.

Breathing out, I feel solid.

Breathing in, I see myself as still water.

Breathing out, I reflect things as they are.

Breathing in, I see myself as space.

Breathing out, I feel free.

Each duet of inhalation and exhalation is meant to be
repeated about ten times, until you feel calm and centered.
Then you move on to the next duet.

Another meditation from the Navajo Indians is
simply:

Before me peaceful
Behind me peaceful
Under me peaceful
Over me peaceful
Around me peaceful.

You can repeat this silently or out loud as you meditate.

Once you are relaxed into meditation, you can add techniques such as autosuggestion and visualization. You can also explore your body with a technique I call "inner gazing." Concentrate your awareness on any part of your body that is uncomfortable. Explore the tension you might be holding in your diaphragm muscles and your shoulders (asthmatics tend to hold their shoulders hunched and high). Experience the discomfort, and then consciously relax your tense muscles in that area.

SELF-HYPNOSIS

The word *hypnosis* comes from the name of the Greek god of sleep, Hypnos. Indeed, hypnotizability seems linked to the rapid eye movement (REM) sleep that occurs during dreaming. It appears that highly hypnotizable individuals can visualize images so clearly and in such detail that they are almost like hallucinations or home movies—the kind of images generated during dreams. They also seem to have a talent for what has been called "lucid dreaming," the ability to "dream" while awake and conscious. In lucid dreaming, subjects control and direct the subject matter of waking visions.

Hypnosis can be a powerful tool to alleviate stress, and it can include autosuggestions that reprogram the mind and body. Under hypnosis, certain individuals have been able to produce anesthesia in any part of their body. In fact, at one time this technique was so popular that in Nancy, France, it was used on more than thirty thousand patients in the late 1800s. Posthypnotic suggestions to improve sleep, control pain, and quit addictive behavior like smoking can be effective. Bleeding can be controlled under hypnosis. In fact, when injured or in shock from extreme stress, we instantly enter a kind of hypnotic state where our movement, breathing, and bleeding are slowed.

Randi, a twenty-three-year-old patient of mine, found she could not meditate on her own. She felt uncomfortable and simply couldn't concentrate. Her wheezing as well as emotional anxieties made it hard for her to sit still. She was, however, open to the idea of hypnosis. After learning simple relaxation and meditation techniques, where she relaxed her entire body part by part, I guided her into a hypnotic trance and gave her a series of suggestions that her lungs would become open and she would feel warmth through her entire chest area. Her response during each training session in the office was excellent, but even so, Randi had trouble practicing on her own. Our solution was to tape one of our office sessions, so that she could practice at home. A year later, she still uses the tape daily.

Surprisingly, you can obtain significant effects from hypnosis after just a few days of practice. I suggest to patients that they use self-hypnosis in two ways: to ameliorate physical discomfort and to trace back a symptom or flare-up to a particular precipitating event or experience.

Here's a simple way to learn self-hypnosis. Sit in a comfortable position in a chair, with legs uncrossed. Place a lit candle before you, and observe the flame. As you observe it, suggest to yourself that your eyelids are feeling heavier and heavier, almost heavy enough to close. Heavier and heavier. As you feel them close, say a phrase to yourself, such as "Relax now." Or pick a key word that has meaning for you: perhaps the beautiful island where you spent a romantic weekend, a color that you feel is relaxing, or a word like "Om" or "Peace." (After you have practiced self-hypnosis for a while, your body will respond with instant relaxation to the word alone.)

Breathe deeply and slowly.

Now, as your eyes are closed, consciously tighten and then relax each of your muscles. Start with your face: scrunch it up, then relax. Follow this procedure with your neck, shoulders, forearms, biceps, triceps, your chest, stomach, lower back, buttocks, thighs, calves, toes.

Continue to breathe deeply. Your body should feel heavy, like a sandbag. Suggest to yourself that you are going deeper and deeper into a state of peace, comfort, drowsiness, safety, relaxation. Count back slowly from ten to zero as you descend into ever deeper planes of relaxation. Count again from ten to zero, and again, until you feel utterly and totally relaxed. If you wish, pause at each number and say something relaxing: "Ten . . . I am becoming relaxed and open to suggestion. Nine . . . I will soon be in a deep, relaxed trance. Eight . . . with each count, I am becoming more relaxed and receptive. Seven . . . with each breath, I am releasing tension, and my entire body is coming to a state of deep rest, comfort, and peace. Six . . . with each count, I am going deeper. . . ."

Allow about twenty minutes to enter this state of hypnotic trance the first few times. If you want to test whether you are in a hypnotic trance, you can try a few different methods:

- Suggest to yourself that your eyelids are glued shut. Imagine the glue spread thickly on them. Count to three. Try to open your lids on the count of three. If you feel unable to open them, you are in a hypnotic trance.
- Try to make part of your body numb. Suggest to yourself, for instance, that your arm feels numb, as if you had just slept on it. Imagine the skin on your arm feeling as thick as your mouth does when the dentist gives you a shot of novocaine. If your arm feels that numb, you have successfully achieved a hypnotic trance.

Once you are in this state, you can give yourself hypnotic suggestions. They might be, "My lungs are being healed. They are being bathed in soothing white light. Pure, healing oxygen is filling every part of my lungs. Each cell is being healed completely."

In general, autosuggestions should be direct, concrete, and simple, and they should always be phrased positively. Don't say: "My lungs will stop wheezing now." Say: "My lungs are opening up and relaxing now." Try to keep all suggestions in the present tense. Autosuggestion works well with visualization.

A variant on hypnosis and autosuggestion, called "autogenic modification," was developed by Dr. Johannes Schultz, a Berlin psychiatrist. He taught a form of hypnosis in which one relaxed in a comfortable position and suggested to oneself that warmth and heaviness were filling the body. This was combined with yoga techniques and special exercises designed to help specific programs. For asthma, he suggested the phrase "It breathes me, it breathes me calm and regular." To enhance and deepen respiration, he suggested the phrase "My heartbeat is calm and regular. It breathes me."

I find autogenic suggestions helpful when patients have developed a new symptom, such as anxiety in response to a crisis or a persistent cough after a bout of bronchitis. In such cases, self-hypnosis along with positive suggestions can help one over a difficult time.

VISUALIZATION

Vision is our most powerful sense, and visualization has long been known to be one of our most powerful mind-body techniques, one that can measurably alter the immune system. According to fascinating new research at Harvard University by Dr. Stephen Kosslyn, the same brain centers are stimulated whether we actually see something or merely visualize it in our imagination. That means that when we visualize or imagine something, the brain cells receive signals as if the picture were really happening. That may be why our body tends to respond to vivid mental imagery as if the images were really true.

Dr. Edmund Jacobson, a physiologist, asked individuals to visualize themselves running. He then measured their muscular contractions and found they were exactly like those that would have been produced if the volunteers were actually running.

In another famous study, boys were divided into three groups and tested on their ability to shoot basketball free throws. Then one group practiced shooting the free throws every day; a second group visualized themselves shooting free throws, and a third group didn't practice or visualize. The groups that visualized or practiced improved markedly.

According to psychiatrist Dr. Gerald Epstein, author of *Healing into Immortality*, visualization works well in asthma. Dr. Epstein is conducting a study of visualization and asthma for the National Institutes of Health, and as Dr. Epstein points out, the process requires commitment and practice at visualizing. Potential patients are tested by being asked if they can imagine a table with a box of flat balloons of many different colors, and then if they can imagine taking some of the balloons and blowing them up. If you can visualize this, you may be an excellent candidate for this type of mind-body technique.

"One patient," recalled Dr. Epstein, in an interview with me, "came in with peak flow meter readings of two hundred and got them up to seven hundred just by visualizing. Another student of mine had been asthmatic most of her thirty-five years, and with two sessions of imagery and one session of talking she was completely free of her asthma. Another woman who was in her sixties and had suffered from asthma for ten years was able to stop taking her medications after visualization."

Pain centers and cancer clinics throughout the country utilize visualization techniques. Dr. O. Carl Simonton, a popularizer of visualization in cancer, counsels patients to visualize white blood cells as a vast army, powerful polar bears, or white sharks devouring cancer cells. Studies of his patients have found that the visualizers live twice as long after the diagnosis of cancer as the nonvisualizers.

Visualization can accompany meditation or self-hypnosis. In fact, it is most effective when you are in a deeply relaxed state. My favorite visualization for asthma patients is one mentioned earlier in this chapter: imagine yourself on a beach, with crystal skies and water, and a cool breeze. (I choose the beach because most asthmatics feel better near the ocean. There is no pollen, no dust, very few allergens. The wind and the humidity are good for the lungs.) Indulge your visualization of this wonderful beach, with sweeping white sands, and the deep crystalline blue of the waters. Embellish your vision. Then imagine a perfect white sailboat. Get in the boat. As you breathe out, you blow the sails. They billow and fill with air. The sailboat moves rapidly along. Relax, and it slows. Blow the sails, and the boat moves. Feel the warm, healing sun all over your body, especially your chest and lungs. Feel the soothing salt spray, the wind in your face. Feel your entire body expanding and healing in response to the sun and sea.

Serita, a fifty-six-year-old secretary in a nursing home, found that visualization helped her a great deal. She often felt anxious and tense when dealing with patients who were suffering from mental and physical debility. In addition, some of her coworkers liked to smoke and that bothered her. She began to practice a visualization in which she imagined herself on a cruise with her family that she had actually gone on the year before. In her visualization, she looked out on water all around her and imagined cool breezes. She felt her lungs opening.

For another patient who frequently suffered from bronchial infections, I recommended visualizing her immune system attacking the bacteria every day. She pictured the vitamins she was taking being absorbed into her cells, so that her cells could destroy invading microorganisms. This visualization was highly effective.

One particularly nice meditation involves a ball of light. With your eyes closed, reach out in front of you and catch hold of an imaginary ball in your hands. Bring the ball close to you, and imagine that it is transformed into brilliant white light—transparent, luminous, and healing. As you breathe, feel this ball of light float out of your hands and come to rest at the center of your chest. Let your attention rest on this healing sphere of white light.

An effective visualization for combating stress is known as the "hollow body" meditation. This exercise seems to reduce pain and to calm the neuromuscular system. Sit comfortably, and bring your attention to your breath. As you inhale, imagine your breath as a luminous white mist that completely fills your head. Breathe out, and as you do, imagine your head as open space. Breathe in, and draw luminous white mist into your neck and throat. Breathe out, leaving only open space in your neck and throat. Continue with every part of your body—your shoulders, chest, stomach, arms, hands, legs, feet. Each time you breathe out the luminous mist, imagine that this particular part of your body is completely open. If you find that a certain area seems dense or solid, and you cannot experience it as open, imagine that you are cleaning out that area with a laser beam sweeping from top to bottom, front to back, and in spirals.

Once you have cleared out your entire body with luminous mist and left it open and hollow, allow yourself to feel completely open to a luminous, airy body. Now imagine your body expanding to fill the universe.

BIOFEEDBACK

Yogi adepts in India have been said to spend a lifetime mastering conscious control over the involuntary processes in their body—to the point where they could slow their heart rate and metabolism and survive days of burial or months of fasting. By meditating and becoming acutely aware of the most subtle signals of biological functions like heart rate and metabolism, these yogis were able to perform remarkable feats.

We may not want to practice being buried alive for days at a time, but today biofeedback, using instruments to help you become aware of processes in your body, is an accepted medical therapy. Modern medical technology now makes it possible for us to tune into the incredibly subtle signals of involuntary processes in our body. These processes are usually regulated by the autonomic nervous system, which controls the heart, blood vessels, hormonal secretions, and other functions. Once you receive feedback about these processes, you can learn to bring them under your voluntary control.

Biofeedback machines give you information about muscle tension, skin temperature and resistance, brain wave activity, blood pressure, heart rate, and blood flow. Biofeedback training teaches you to be newly attuned to signs of stress and tension that you had never before noticed, and to offset your body's alarm response.

The practical application of biofeedback was pioneered by Alyce and Elmer Green of the Menninger Foundation, in the 1960s. In one fascinating experiment, the Greens invited a yogi adept, Swami Rama, to their laboratory. The yogi was wired to sensors and repeatedly performed the astonishing feat of consciously altering his blood flow so that one part of his palm was nearly 17 degrees warmer than an area a few inches away. A university student who heard about the experiment decided to try to accomplish the same feat using biofeedback. Within two weeks, he had succeeded.

Since that time biofeedback has become an accepted treatment for many stress-related illnesses, from migraine headaches to colitis, muscle pain, and yes, asthma. Recently, biofeedback has been used to help epileptics control seizures and to help cancer patients boost their immune systems. Even the firing of nerve cells in the brain can be controlled by biofeedback. One researcher, John Basmajian, trained subjects by sounding a drum each time a specific neuron in their brain fired. They quickly learned how to control the rhythm of that firing, creating drumrolls and varying beats.

In my practice I use biofeedback, employing computer-driven programs that measure brain waves, breathing, body heat, sweat, and other parameters and give feedback to the patient to help them establish regular breathing patterns in a relaxed state of mind. Biofeedback practitioners use various monitoring devices—usually with electrodes—that transform body signals into auditory or visual signs, such as sounds, flickering or flashing lights, or needle readings on a meter. The basic types of biofeedback include the following:

- EMG (electromyogram). This monitors muscle tension, most commonly in the muscles in your forehead, jaw, and shoulders, which are the ones most responsive to stress. However, this type of training has also been used in a wide variety of other applications, including pelvic muscle training for women who are suffering from incontinence or pelvic pain.
- Temperature. A thermograph, a temperature-sensitive monitor, records fluctuations in body temperature. The thermograph monitors finger, hand, or foot temperature through a heat sensor. Skin temperature decreases whenever you are anxious, because capillaries in your skin constrict and limit blood flow. By raising your skin tem-

perature, you can create an anti-stress, anti-anxiety effect. This kind of training has been quite successful with migraine headaches, as well as cold hands and feet. In general, it's a good indication of whether you are relaxed or not.

- GSR (galvanic skin response). A dermograph measures the electrical resistance in your skin. The lower the measurable voltage, the lower your emotional arousal. (GSR has been used in lie detector tests.) This kind of biofeedback is very useful in phobias and anxiety states.
- EEG (electroencephalogram). This is perhaps the most common method of biofeedback, which measures brain waves. Brain waves fall into four ranges: beta (wide awake), alpha (relaxed), theta (deep reverie, trance, or light sleep), and delta (deep sleep).

Many insurance companies will cover biofeedback training, and within a few sessions, one will see results. Some machines can be rented or bought for home use and are relatively inexpensive. I myself particularly enjoy a biofeedback device called the Breathwork Explorer, which I also mentioned in chapter 10.

As soon as I try this machine, which gives you light and sound feedback when you breathe deeply and slowly, I feel myself relaxing. My breathing immediately gets easier. I feel as if I am listening to the sound of waves crashing on the shoreline in Montauk. I can visualize myself on the beach at night in the summer, and my breathing controls the sound of the waves. I inhale and exhale fully, listening to the sound of waves and then the sound of silence. It is an extremely effective and ingenious biofeedback device.

Software made for personal computers can provide you with home systems that are both effective and cost-conscious. Biofeedback devices range from about $60 for the GSR 2 Biofeedback System, a handheld galvanic skin response device, to the BE-200 Brain Exercise, an electroencephalographic training device that links up to an IBM-compatible computer and costs about $1,600.

The second type of device is extremely beneficial and has been used to treat patients suffering from hyperactivity (attention deficit disorder) as well as premenstrual syndrome, anxiety, and depression. In different "games," you learn, for instance, to manipulate a balloon, making it rise above a certain line. The balloon only rises when your brain waves produce a certain pattern. You can train yourself to shift brain states at will, without drugs. By shifting into profoundly relaxed or clear-and-alert states, you can modify your entire mind-body condition. These devices are obviously too expensive for most individuals to use at home, but as computer technology evolves, their prices will come down. At present, they are used by practitioners throughout the country.

HEALING THROUGH SOUND AND BRAIN SYNCHRONY

According to French physician, psychologist, and ear specialist Dr. Alfred A. Tomatis, one function of the ear is to charge the brain with electrical potential, through the vibration of sound. Tomatis believes that people have chanted for thousands of years not only because they considered chants sacred, but because the chanting itself has physiological effects. Certain sounds can charge the brain, and in many cases, meditating can be greatly enhanced by chanting and/or sound because it gives the brain the stimulus it craves, while focusing and quieting the mind.

The music of Mozart has been shown, in various studies, to be both relaxing and energizing. At the University of Chicago, music was introduced to alleviate the tension of patients undergoing surgery, and this practice has turned out to be so successful that music was introduced into six major operating rooms at the Nathan Goldblatt Memorial Hospital.

Mark Ryder, Ph.D., of Southern Methodist University, found that individuals who listened to the music of the Harmonic Choir showed decreased heart rate, respiration, and galvanic skin response. Dr. Herbert Benson, a Harvard psychiatrist who studied the effects of meditation (or the relaxation response, as he called it) discovered that when people repeated a single word, or mantra, there was a decrease in oxygen consumption, heartbeat, pulse rate, and the rate of metabolism. There was also an increase in alpha waves.

Relaxation audiotapes or CDs played on your portable stereo unit can help facilitate deeply relaxed states. These recordings utilize "binaural beats," a special combination of subliminal rhythms and beats that entrain brain waves in the alpha and theta ranges, which are associated with relaxation and trance states, respectively. "Light and sound" machines, which include headphones and goggles, are also available; these devices allow you to relax to music and flashing lights that entrain brain waves. This technology cannot force you to relax if you don't want to. It simply facilitates meditation, much like training wheels on a bicycle. Recordings and light and sound machines are available in many popular catalogues and in big bookstore and audio chains, and they are advertised in magazines like *Omni* and *Psychology Today*. I also record relaxation tapes for my patients and have had excellent, even transformational, results.

Sound can be a valuable adjunct to any kind of meditation or visualization.

YOGA

Yoga is a uniquely holistic therapy for asthma patients, one that combines proper breathing techniques with relaxing postures that increase circulation, flexibility, and strength. Most yoga sessions end with a period of meditation and relaxation. Therefore, I consider yoga the ideal mind-body technique.

Studies of patients at the Yoga Institute of Bombay found that in asthmatics who'd had years of orthodox medical treatment, training in yoga techniques led to significant improvement. A 1986 study in *Journal of Asthma* reported on 53 patients with asthma who studied yoga for two weeks, learning breathing, breath slowing techniques, physical postures, and meditation. They practiced yoga for an hour each day and were compared to a control group of 53 asthmatics. Yoga significantly improved asthma, lessening frequency of attacks, increasing peak flow scores, and reducing drug intake. Another study found that 570 asthmatics who practiced yoga were able to reduce medication to a remarkable degree; and similar studies with follow-ups of two years found that improvement from yoga lasts.

There are different types of yoga practiced in this country. The most common, known as hatha yoga, focuses on various postures and stretches. A few that are particularly beneficial in asthma include the well-known Salute to the Sun, with which most yoga classes begin. This exercise, if done rigorously, can be truly aerobic, and also stretches the entire body. Other excellent postures for asthma include the Cobra, which stretches and expands the entire chest area, and the Fish, which also opens and stretches the chest, shoulders, and neck.

Another form of yoga that is also popular is kundalini yoga, which involves breathing and chanting in an attempt to circulate energy from the base of the spine throughout the body. This yoga is well-known in the literature for being extremely potent, and there are even occasional warnings against practicing it alone without guidance.

Simple yoga postures are not difficult to learn. Inexpensive classes are usually available at local gyms and YMCAs; books and videos can be highly instructive and can help you to learn and practice yoga on your own. One fifty-five-year-old patient of mine complained that she could not exercise because her muscles were too sore and her breathing too labored. When she began to practice yoga, she soon found it was an excellent way to tone her body and to learn to breathe properly. In each movement in yoga, one must take a complete breath (inhalation and exhalation). Now yoga has become part of her daily routine.

TAI CHI AND CHI GUNG

Like yoga, these Eastern forms of exercise pay attention to breathing, relaxation, and energy flow throughout the entire body. There are some amazing and true stories of remarkable recoveries not only from asthma but even from cystic fibrosis with dedicated practice of chi gung. According to Kumar Frantzis, author of *Opening the Energy Gates of Your Body,* practice of chi gung saved him from death. Frantzis had contracted an extremely virulent form of hepatitis in India, a form which killed two close friends but which he survived.

Chi gung literally means "energy work." It is reputed to give a feeling of relaxed power, to balance and strengthen internal organs, and to improve vascular function. For instance, chi gung exercises do not work to strengthen the heart but to increase the elasticity of blood vessels, so the heart does not need to pump as hard. Best of all for the asthmatic, it involves slow, deep, regular breathing and movement that bring oxygen deep into the tissues.

Tai chi is similar to chi gung, although it is a quieter

form of exercise with great attention to slow movement, postures, and internal states.

Both can be quite beneficial in asthma. A seventy-five-year-old patient of mine truly enjoys tai chi because it requires very slow movements tied to deep breathing. She feels more limber and active, and her lungs are less congested since she began practicing this form of exercise.

ACUPUNCTURE

Well over four thousand years old, acupuncture is one of the oldest forms of healing known to man. It originated in China and is still being practiced today throughout the world. Acupuncture has demonstrated statistically significant effects upon a wide range of symptoms. It is particularly valuable in stress-related illnesses.

Traditional Chinese medicine views our vital force, or "chi," as the crucial element in health. Chi, according to this view, circulates through pathways in the body that are called meridians. Each meridian feeds a main organ or function of the body, such as the heart, kidneys, lungs, colon, and so forth. When the vital chi energy is flowing freely and harmoniously through all twelve meridians, one is in perfect health. When the energy is out of balance, blocked, or excessive, ill health results. Acupuncture attempts to correct imbalances and reestablish a harmonious flow, by directing energy at special points located on the meridians. When needles are gently inserted into these points (and sometimes twirled or heated), energy is either drawn to a meridian or dispersed from it.

Any practitioner of acupuncture views the body, mind, and spirit as a whole. An acupuncturist looks upon symptoms as an indication of trouble but not as the actual trouble itself.

When choosing an acupuncturist, it's best to seek out an

experienced practitioner who has at least five years of clinical experience. A medical doctor who has had a "course" in acupuncture but who still practices primarily Western medicine may not fully understand the real art of this healing practice.

OSTEOPATHIC MANIPULATION

I am an osteopathic physician, and utilize osteopathic manipulation in my practice every day and find it to be invaluable. Osteopathy was begun almost one hundred years ago by Dr. Andrew Taylor Still, an M.D. who found that manipulation of joints, muscles, and tendons could benefit many health problems. This modality can help in certain cases of asthma, because spinal manipulations can relieve muscular tension in the chest and restore proper nerve flow to the lungs. As far back as 1925, studies of osteopathic manipulation in asthma showed patients obtained relief and had half as many asthmatic attacks with regular treatments. Other studies have demonstrated improvement in oxygen levels, total lung capacity, and ability of the lungs to work. A 1982 study of this type of therapy found that respiratory infections were significantly reduced in one hundred patients who received osteopathy.

Osteopathic manipulation (and its close cousin, chiropractic) can be an essential part of a treatment plan for an asthmatic whose lungs are already compromised. This type of treatment can help increase the flow of information between the muscular and nervous systems, reducing blockages and imbalances.

This technique also offers specific adjustments for lymphatic drainage. The lymph system is known to drain in specific channels, especially in an area in front of the chest known as the thoracic duct. You can actually help move the lymph along if it becomes blocked, so that your body can cleanse itself of toxins. I know of one patient who came into the hospital with pneumonia so severe she was expected to die during the night. An osteopathic physician stayed with her the entire night performing lymphatic drainage techniques, and by morning she was much better.

SLEEP

It may seem odd to include sleep in a chapter on mind-body medicine, as if sleep were an activity that could be "performed," but new research suggests that getting to bed on time and sleeping properly is much more important to long-term health than was formerly thought. Patients with asthma, as you who are reading this book probably know well, suffer terribly with sleep disturbances.

"Sleep is a vital physiological need, like food and water," stated Mark Rosekind, a researcher at NASA. Lack of sleep can accelerate aging and suppress the immune system. The average person needs eight to nine hours of sleep a night and gets only seven. Only 10 percent of the population needs less than eight hours of sleep.

Perhaps the greatest impact of sleep deprivation is on the immune system: levels of interleukin-1, an important organizer of the immune response, rise when a person sleeps. Lack of sleep erodes the body's nightly work of repairing damage. Important chemicals are released during sleep, like human growth hormone, which helps the body restore itself.

Asthmatics suffer from sleep disturbance in part because of innate biological or circadian rhythms. Patients with asthma consistently have high levels of adrenaline in their blood during the day and low levels at night. Adrenaline is a natural bronchodilator. In addition, levels of antiinflammatory cortisol are higher during the day than at night (except for patients taking steroids). Asthmatics' airways produce more inflammatory cells such as eosinophils and neutrophils at night than during the day. This means that asthmatics often wake at night with tight, wheezing lungs and a general feeling of discomfort.

There are several ways to enhance your ability to get a good night's sleep. One substance of great interest is melatonin, a hormone that is released by the pineal gland, a tiny light-sensitive gland in your brain. During daylight, melatonin production is suppressed. At night, it is released. A dose of melatonin an hour before bedtime can help ensure a more restful night's sleep.

Herbs such as valerian, chamomile, passion flower, and hops can also aid sleep. In addition, branched chain amino acids, which are available in your health food store, can help by providing the body with precursors of the neurotransmitters that aid sleep.

Daily exercise can also help regulate the body and increase the ability to sleep. Deep-breathing techniques and meditation used nightly can be of aid. Sleep is important, and it should not be overlooked.

COGNITIVE REFRAMING

Stress can be reframed as challenge, and that simple shift in perspective can have a profound influence on healing. In particular, if an asthmatic utilizes his or her preferred relaxation technique (whether it be meditation, breathwork, hypnosis, or any of the other techniques surveyed in this chapter) along with a heightened awareness of the cues that signal the beginning of an attack, he or she can learn to convert symptoms into signals for self-healing. The symptom is no longer an early warning sign of a painful attack but a signal to begin using the techniques that truly can avert an attack.

Cognitive reframing works because of actual physiological changes produced during the perception of stress in contrast to the perception of challenge. Studies in the early 1980s found a fascinating distinction between negative and positive emotions in response to stress. The body's response to threat (stress) is associated with:

1. an increase in the blood level of chemicals called catecholamines—specifically epinephrine and norepinephrine
2. the release of cortisol from the adrenal cortex into the bloodstream

A chronic response to stress leads to chronic elevations of norepinephrine and cortisol—and a compromised immune system. Norepinephrine, for instance, blocks the ability of white blood cells to kill tumor cells. In addition, higher levels of cortisol can be linked with depressed immune function, especially when stress is chronic.

Challenge, or good stress, causes the release of catecholamines only. Most interesting of all, however, studies of coping skills found that the greater a patient's sense of being able to cope, the lower the level of catecholamines.

If stress can be converted into challenge, and that challenge can be seen as surmountable, the healing impact on the body will be significant. According to research by Suzanne Kobasa and Salvatore Maddi, at the University of Chicago, those individuals who view stress as a challenge, and change as an opportunity for growth, have little physical reaction to stress. These individuals have far fewer illnesses than those people who see stress as uncontrollable, and change as a threat to the status quo. Psychological hardiness translates into physical hardiness.

Reframing stress as challenge can be done consciously during meditation or hypnosis. According to Ernest Rossi, Ph.D., author of *The Psychobiology of Mind-Body Healing,* "tuning into a symptom with an attitude of respectful inquiry rather than the usual patient stance of avoidance, resistance, and rejection is the first step." Rossi suggests to his patients that their attitude toward their symptoms is very important. "Your symptom or problem is actually your friend! Your symptom is a signal that a creative change is needed in your life."

Rossi suggests transforming a problem into a creative opportunity in this way:

1. Access the circumstances during which a chronic problem becomes manifest. In the case of asthma, this means understanding and reviewing the conditions that usually lead to an attack. Scan these conditions with a kind of internal "radar" so that you can identify each of the triggers of an attack. Now "feel" and sense those triggers. Try to heighten your awareness of those triggers.

2. Use your heightened sensitivity as a radar to scan the minimal cues that might evoke your problem (in this case, an asthma attack). See, hear, feel, intuit your mind-body responses.

3. Recognize and review your usual, painful way of dealing with an asthma attack. Now imagine how your new sensitivity to milder signals can become a resource for problem solving. For instance, you might begin to meditate or visualize the moment a milder signal is present.

See yourself as capable of coping with your asthma. You can scan mild symptoms and environmental triggers, convert them into signals, and use any of the techniques in this chapter to cope effectively with a possible attack. In many cases, you can prevent it from happening. What you once regarded as uncontrollable stress (which released stress hormones and set off a cascade of unpleasant responses in your body) becomes a challenge. Each time you meet that challenge, you feel hope, joy, triumph, and a sense of efficacy. The long-term effect on your immune system can only be remarkably beneficial.

This book began with my personal story, and I am concluding it with this essential information on cognitive reframing because I feel it was this approach that changed my life. When you decide that you are going to treat an illness as a challenge, when your healing becomes a goal you are determined to accomplish and to which you are committed, you move instantly away from the framework of "I've been sick a week, a month, a year. . . . I am never going to get well." Imagine a great baseball player who, when he was a minor league rookie, said to himself, "I haven't batted four hundred this week, I might as well give up." Your health does not need to become a full-time occupation, but you do need to devote yourself to a comprehensive effort at healing your body. I believe that the first step is in the mind.

In your healing process, you will find yourself enjoying triumphs and then suffering setbacks. An emotional crisis or physical stress may set off a bout of bronchitis after months of improvement. An encounter with environmental toxins or allergens, holidays spent at a family home where there are pets, or perhaps your own (very human) tendency to stop being vigilant about practicing CAP once you feel better, may lead to setbacks or temporary relapses. Whenever you are confronted with the challenge du jour, it is important to examine it for information it can give you about your health and how to improve it.

It's especially important to keep your own inner sense of your accomplishments and healing. Sometimes people who do not suffer from a chronic illness have little understanding of the nature and tenacity of such a condition. They may say: "It's been a month already and you're not well." It's important to be clear with your family and friends about the commitment you have to your healing over the long term. I've found that patients must communicate clearly about their needs—for instance, telling a friend or lover that you are allergic to his or her cat and that adjustments will need to be made in the relationship as a result (perhaps having an air filter installed in the nonallergic person's apartment, washing and vacuuming of the problem area, keeping certain rooms pet-free, especially the bedroom). When you are clear in your communication, people who care about you will be willing to work with you, but the important first step is your attitude: determination, commitment, and clarity.

Here's how a patient of mine recently put it:

> On Monday I was on 60 milligrams of prednisone, as I had been for the past four months. And I had my usual feeling of despair over the need to take so much medication, especially when the side effects were beginning to show. I was suffering from acne and weight gain. On Wednesday, however, after our appointment, I was on the exact same amount of medicine and the world had just clocked one more day, but I felt differently. My brain said, "You're going to be okay." It changed the whole complexion of my situation. It was very liberating. I was going to do it. I was going to get well. Nothing was going to get in the way of my getting better and now I was just going to focus on what I needed to do to get healthy. Nothing in my outer life had changed, but I felt different. That was two years ago. Dr. Firshein, you were right!

Today, she is off medication.

All the tools you need are in this book.

DOCTOR'S RECOMMENDATIONS FOR ACTION

1. Recognize that the mind and body have the potential to influence each other, because the brain and immune sys-

tem speak the same chemical language. Mind-body approaches to healing can be a significant step toward healing your asthma.

2. Know that there are many different mind-body approaches. Be willing to experiment with them to find what technique or combination of techniques best suits you. Investigate the following:

- meditation, which includes such popular forms as one-pointed meditation, breath counting, chanting, and open-focus meditation (or mindfulness)
- self-hypnosis
- autogenic modification and autosuggestion
- visualization techniques
- biofeedback, using electromyograms, temperature readings, galvanic skin response, and electroencephalograms (relatively inexpensive biofeedback devices are available for home use)

APPENDIX

American Academy of Allergy, Asthma and Immunology
611 East Wells Street
Milwaukee, WI 53202
1-800-822-2762

American Academy of Environmental Medicine
10 East Randolph Street
New Hope, PA 18938
215-862-4574, 800-LET-HEAL

American College for Advancement in Medicine
23121 Vertugo Drive, Suite 204
Laguna Hills, CA 92653
1-714-583-7666

American College of Allergy, Asthma and Immunology
1645 Oakton Avenue
Des Plaines, IL 60018
1-800-842-7777

American College of Occupational and Environmental
  Medicine
55 West Seegers Road
Arlington Heights, IL 60005
1-847-228-6850

American Environmental Health Center
8345 Walnut Hill Lane, Suite 205
Dallas, TX 75231
1-214-368-4132

American Holistic Medical Association
4101 Lake Boone Trail, Suite 201
Raleigh, NC 27607
1-919-787-5146

American Osteopathic Association
142 East Ontario Street
Chicago, IL 60611
1-800-621-1773

Association for Applied Psychophysiology and Biofeedback
10200 W. 44th Avenue, Suite 304
Wheat Ridge, CO 80033
1-303-422-8436

The Asthma and Allergy Foundation of America
1125 15th Street NW, Suite 502
Washington, DC 20005
1-800-7-ASTHMA

Bastyr University—Natural Health Clinic
14500 Juanita Drive NE
Bothel, WA 98011
1-206-823-1300

Heimlich Institute Foundation, Inc.
2368 Victory Parkway, Suite 410
Cincinnati, OH 45206
1-513-221-0002

Sorvino Asthma Foundation
246 Lafayette Street
New York, NY 10012
212-941-8686

University of Arizona Program in Integrative Medicine
1501 N. Campbell Avenue
P.O. Box 245099
Tucson, AZ 85724-5099
1-520-626-5077

SELECTED NOTES AND REFERENCES

FREE RADICAL DAMAGE, ANTIOXIDANTS AND ASTHMA

Research into the suspected role of free radical damage and antioxidants in asthma continues to grow. Free radicals are reactive oxygen molecules that can cause tissue damage and are markers for inflammation in the body.

Free Radicals

Chanez, P., Dent, G., et al. "Generation of oxygen free radicals from blood eosinophils from asthma patients after stimulation with PAF or phorbol ester." *European Respiratory Journal* (October 1990), 3(9):1002–07.

Chilvers, E. R., Garratt, H., Whyte, M. K., Fink, R., Ind, P. W. "Absence of circulating products of oxygen derived free radicals in acute severe asthma." *European Respiratory Journal* (November 1989), 2(10):950–54.

Cluzel, M., Damon, M., Chanez, P., Bousquet, J., Crastes de Paulet, A., Michel, F. B., Godard, P. "Enhanced alveolar cell luminol-dependent chemiluminescence in asthma." *Journal of Allergy and Clinical Immunology* (August 1987), 80(2):195–201.

Doelman, C. J., Bast, A. "Oxygen radicals in lung pathology." *Free Radical Biology and Medicine* (1990), (5):381–400.

Godard, P., Damon, M., Cluzel, M., Bousquet, J., Chanez, P., Crastes de Paulet, A., Michel, F. B. "Radicaux libres de l'oxygène et asthme bronchique" (Oxygen-free radicals and bronchial asthma). *Allergie et Immunologie* (Paris) (October 1987), 19 (8 Suppl.):15–18.

Kanazawa, H., Kurihara, N., et al. "The role of free radicals in airway obstruction in asthmatic patients." *Chest* (November 1991), 100(5):1319–22.

Kato, M., Morikawa, A., et al. "Effects of antiasthma drugs on superoxide anion generation from human polymorphonuclear leukocytes or hypoxanthine-xanthine oxidase system." *Internal Archives of Allergy and Applied Immunology* (1991), 96(2):128–33.

Levine, Stephen A., and Kidd, Parris M. *Antioxidant Adaptation: Its Role in Free Radical Pathology.* 2nd printing, revised. San Leandro, CA: Biocurrents Division, Allergy Research Group, 1986.

Novak, Z., Nemeth, I., Gyurkovits, K., Varga, S. I., Matkovics, B. "Examination of the role of oxygen free radicals in bronchial asthma in childhood." *Clinica Chimica Acta* (Sept. 30, 1991), 201(3):247–51.

Owen, S., Pearson, D., Suarez-Mendez, V., O'Driscoll, R., Woodcock, A. "Evidence of free-radical activity in asthma" (letter). *New England Journal of Medicine* (Aug. 22, 1991), 325(8):586–87.

Shichijo, T., Ariyama, A., Tsuji, Y. "Oxygen radicals." *Nippon Rinsho. Japanese Journal of Clinical Medicine* (March 1993), 51(3):638–42.

Weiss, E. B. "Toxic oxygen products alter calcium homeostasis in an asthma model." *Journal of Allergy and Clinical Immunology* (June 1985), 75(6):692–97.

Antioxidants

Aderele, W. I., Ette, S. I., Oduwole, O., Ikpeme, S. J. "Plasma vitamin C (ascorbic acid) levels in asthmatic children." *African Journal of Medicine and Medical Sciences* (September–December 1985), 114(3–4):115–20.

Ahlrot-Westerlund, B., Norrby, A. Remarkable success of antioxidant treatment (selenomethionine and vitamin E) to a 34-year-old patient with posterior subcapsular cataract, keratoconus, severe atopic eczema, and asthma (letter). *Acta Ophthalmol* (Copenhagen) (April 1988), 66(2):237–38.

Boljevic, S., Daniljak, I. G., Kogan, A. H. "Changes in free radicals and possibility of their correction in patients with bronchial asthma." *Vojnosanit Pregl* (January–February 1993), 50(1):3–18 (published in Serbo-Croatian, Roman and Russian).

Burgess, C. D., Bremner, P., Thomson, C. D., Crane, J., Siebers, R. W., Beasley, R. "Nebulized beta 2-adrenoceptor agonists do not affect plasma selenium or glutathione peroxidase activity in patients with asthma." *International Journal of Clinical Pharmacology and Therapeutics* (June 1994), 32(6):290–92.

Calhoun, W. J., Bush, R. K. "Enhanced reactive oxygen species metabolism of airspace cells and airway inflammation follow antigen challenge in human asthma." *Journal of Allergy and Clinical Immunology* (September 1990), 86(3 Pt 1):306–13.

De Lucia, F., Bonavia, M., Crimi, E., Scaricabarozzi, I., Brusasco, V. "Antiinflammatory-antioxidant treatment with a methane sulfonanilide in allergen-induced asthma." *Annals of Allergy* (May 1991), 66(5):424–29.

el-Kholy, M. S., Gas Allah, M. A., El-Shimi, S., el-Baz, F., el-Tayeb, H., Abdel-Hamid, M. S. "Zinc and copper status in children with bronchial asthma and atopic dermatitis." *Journal of the Egyptian Public Health Association* (1990), 65(5–6):657–68.

Flatt, A., Pearce, N., Thomson, C. D., Sears, M. R., Robinson, M. F., Beasley, R. "Reduced selenium in asthmatic subjects in New Zealand." *Thorax* (February 1990), 45(2):95–99.

Greene, L. S. "Asthma and oxidant stress: Nutritional, environmental, and genetic risk factors." *Journal of the American College of Nutrition* (August 1995), 14(4):317–24.

Hasselmark, L., Malmgren, R., Unge, G., Zetterstrom, O. "Lowered platelet glutathione peroxidase activity in patients with intrinsic asthma." *Allergy* (October 1990), 45(7):523–27.

Hasselmark, L., Malmgren, R., Zetterstrom, O., Unge, G. "Selenium supplementation in intrinsic asthma." *Allergy* (January 1993), 48(1):30–36.

Hatch, G. E. "Asthma, inhaled oxidants, and dietary antioxidants." *American Journal of Clinical Nutrition* (March 1995), 61(3 Suppl.):625S–630S.

Jarjour, N. N., Calhoun, W. J. "Enhanced production of oxygen radicals in asthma." *Journal of Laboratory and Clinical Medicine* (January 1994), 123(1):131–36.

Lansing, M. W., Mansour, E., Ahmed, A., Cortes, A., Garcia, L., Lauredo, I. T., Wanner, A., Abraham, W. M. "Lipid mediators contribute to oxygen-radical-induced airway responses in sheep." *American Review of Respiratory Disease* (December 1991), 144(6):1291–96.

Malmgren, R., Unge, G., Zetterstrom, O., Theorell, H., de Wahl, K. "Lowered glutathione-peroxidase activity in asthmatic patients with food and aspirin intolerance." *Allergy* (January 1986), 41(1):43–45.

Mohsenin, V., Dubois, A. B., Douglas, J. S. "Effect of ascorbic acid on response to methacholine challenge in asthmatic subjects." *American Review of Respiratory Disease* (February 1983), 127(2):143–47.

Olusi, S. O., Ojutiku, O. O., Jessop, W. J., Iboko, M. I. "Plasma and white blood cell ascorbic acid concentrations in patients with bronchial asthma." *Clinica Chimica Acta* (March 1, 1979), 92(2):161–66.

Pearson, D. J., Suarez-Mendez, V. J., Day, J. P., Miller, P. F. *Clinical and Experimental Allergy* (March 1991), 21(2):203–08.

Plaza, V., Prat, J., Rosello, J., Ballester, E., Ramis, I., Mullol, J., Gelpi, E., Vives-Corrons, J. L., Picado, C. "In vitro release of arachidonic acid metabolites, glutathione peroxidase, and oxygen-free radicals from platelets of asthmatic patients with and without aspirin intolerance." *Thorax* (May 1995), 50(5):490–96.

Powell, C. V., Nash, A. A., Powers, H. J., Primhak, R. A. "Antioxidant status in asthma." (July 1994), *Pediatric Pulmonology* 18(1):34–38.

Sanders, S. P., Zweier, J. L., Harrison, S. J., Trush, M. A., Rembish, S. J., Liu, M. C. "Spontaneous oxygen radical production at sites of antigen challenge in allergic subjects." *American Journal of Respiratory and Critical Care Medicine* (June 1995), 151(6):1725–33.

Schachter, E. N., Schlesinger, A. "The attenuation of exercise-induced bronchospasm by ascorbic acid." *Annals of Allergy* (September 1982), 49(3):146–51.

Smith, L. J., Houston, M., Anderson, J. "Increased levels of glutathione in bronchoalveolar lavage fluid from patients with asthma." *American Review of Respiratory Disease* (June 1993), 147(6 Pt 1):1461–64.

Stone, J., Hinks, L. J., Beasley, R., Holgate, S. T., Clayton, B. A. "Reduced selenium status of patients with asthma." *Clinical Science* (November 1989), 77(5):495–500.

Tarlo, S. M., Sussman, G. L. "Asthma and anaphylactoid reactions to food additives." *Canadian Family Physician* (May 1993), 39:1119–23.

Troisi, R. J., Willett, W. C., Weiss, S. T., Trichopoulos, D., Rosner, B., Speizer, F. E. "A prospective study of diet and adult-onset asthma." *American Journal of Respiratory and Critical Care Medicine* (May 1995), 151(5):1401–08.

Vachier, I., Chanez, P., Le Doucen, C., Damon, M., Descomps, B., Godard, P. "Enhancement of reactive oxygen species formation in stable and unstable asthmatic patients." *European Respiratory Journal* (September 1994), 7(9):1585–92.

Vachier, I., Damon, M., Le Doucen, C., de Paulet, A. C., Chanez, P., Michel, F. B., Godard, P. "Increased oxygen species generation in blood monocytes of asthmatic patients." *American Review of Respiratory Disease* (November 1994), 146(5 Pt 1):1161–66.

Vachier, I., Le Doucen, C., Loubatiere, J., Damon, M., Terouanne, B., Nicolas, J. C., Chanez, P., Godard, P. "Imaging reactive oxygen species in asthma." *Journal of Bioluminescence and Chemiluminescence* (May–June 1994), 9(3):171–75.

FISH OILS, DIETARY OILS, ASTHMA AND INFLAMMATION

The use of fish oils to treat asthma continues to be controversial. It is suspected that they reduce inflammation in a variety of conditions, including arthritis and colitis. They work by reducing the byproducts of inflammation, as well as the mediators of inflammation in the body. In aspirin-sensitive asthmatics, however, they may worsen the condition.

Agrawal, Devendra K., and Townley, Robert G., eds. *Inflammatory Cells and Mediators in Bronchial Asthma*. Boca Raton, FL: CRC Press, 1991.

Arm, J. P., Horton, C. E., Mencia-Huerta, J. M., House, F. Eiser, N. M., Clark, T. J., Spur, B. W., Lee, T. H. "Effect of dietary supplementation with fish oil lipids on mild asthma." *Thorax* (February 1988), 43(2):84–92.

Arm, J. P., Horton, C. E., et al. "The effects of dietary supplementation with fish oil lipids on the airways' response to inhaled allergen in bronchial asthma." *American Review of Respiratory Disease* (June 1989), 139(6):1395–400.

Arm, J. P., Lee, T. H. "The use of fish oil in bronchial asthma." *Allergy Proceedings* (May–June 1989), 10(3):185–87.

Dry, J., Vincent, D. "Effect of a fish oil diet on asthma: Results of a 1-year double-blind study." *International Archives of Allergy and Applied Immunology* (1991), 95(2–3):156–57.

Erasmus, U. *Fats and Oils: The Complete Guide to Fats and Oils in Health and Nutrition*. Burnaby, Vancouver: Alive Books, 1986.

Horrobin, D. F., et al. "Effects of essential fatty acids on prostaglandin biosynthesis." *Biochemistry Acta* 43 (1984), S114–S120.

Knapp, H. R. "Omega-3 fatty acids in respiratory diseases: A review." *Journal of the American College of Nutrition* (February 1995), 14(1):18–23.

Lee, T. H., Arm. J. P., et al. "Effects of dietary fish oil lipids on allergic and inflammatory diseases." *Allergy Proceedings* (September–October 1991), 12(5):299–303.

————. "The Effects of a Fish-Oil Enriched Diet on Experimentally Induced and Clinical Asthma." *Advances in Prostaglandin, Thromboxane, and Leukotriene Research*, Vol. 19, edited by B. Samuelsson, P. Y.-K. Wong, and F. F. Sun. New York: Raven Press, 1989, pp. 606–09.

Picado, C., Castillo, J. A., et al. "Effects of a fish-oil enriched diet on aspirin intolerant asthmatic patients: A pilot study." *Thorax* (February 1988), 43(2):93–97.

Sakai, K., Okuyama, H., Shimazaki, H., Katagiri, M., Torii, S., Matsushita, T., Baba, S. "Fatty acid compositions of plasma lipids in atopic dermatitis/asthma patients." *Arerugi* (1994), 43(1):37–43.

Thien, F. C., Mencia-Huerta, J. M., Lee, T. H. "Dietary fish oil effects on seasonal hay fever and asthma in pollen-sensitive subjects." *American Review of Respiratory Disease* (May 1993), 147(5):1138–43.

SIDE EFFECTS OF DRUGS

Medications can be helpful in emergencies, or as a bridge to overcome acute or chronic asthma. However, these medications come with potentially serious side effects, and ultimately the goal of an asthma treatment program should be to reduce dependence on drugs. There are many studies detailing the harmful side effects of asthma medication, especially cortisone. Here are a selection.

Adinoff, A. D., Hollister, J. R., "Steroid induced fractures and bone loss in patients with asthma." *New England Journal of Medicine* (Aug. 4, 1983), 309(5):265–68.

Bartel, P. R., Ubbink, J. B., Delport, R., Lotz, B. P., Becker, P. J. "Vitamin B-6 supplementation and theophylline-related effects in humans." *American Journal of Clinical Nutrition* (July 1994), 60(1):93–99.

Bien, J. P., Bloom, M. D., Evans, R. L., Specker, B., O'Brien, K. P. "Intravenous theophylline in pediatric status asthamaticus. A prospective, randomized, double-blind, placebo-controlled trial." *Clinical Pediatrics* (September 1995), 34(9):475–81.

Bittar, G., Friedman, H. S. "The arrhythmogenicity of theophylline. A multivariate analysis of clinical determinants." *Chest* (June 1991), 99(6):1415–20.

Carpi, John. "Inhaled albuterol may worsen child's attention-deficit disorder." *Family Practice News* (April 1995), 5.

Chazan, R., Karwat, K., et al. "Cardiac arrhythmias as a result of intravenous infusions of theophylline in patients with airway obstruction." *International Journal of Clinical Pharmacology and Therapeutics* (March 1995), 33(3):170–75.

Decramer, M., Stas, K. J. "Corticosteroid-induced myopathy involving respiratory muscles in patients with chronic obstructive pulmonary disease or asthma." *American Review of Respiratory Disease* (September 1992), 146(3):800–02.

Dunlap, N. E., Bailey, W. C. "Corticosteroids in asthma." *Southern Medical Journal* (April 1990), 83(4):428–32.

Dunn, P. J., Mahood, C. B., et al. "Dehydroepiandrosterone sulphate concentrations in asthmatic patients: Pilot study." *New Zealand Medical Journal* (Nov. 28, 1984), 97(768):850–58.

Edwards, T. B., Dockhorn, R. J., Wagner, D. E., et al. "Efficacy of once daily extended-release theophylline in decreasing the use of inhaled beta 2-agonists in stable, mild-to-moderate asthma patients." *Annals of Allergy, Asthma and Immunology* (November 1995), 75(5):409–16.

Feher, K. G., Koo, E., Feher, T. "Adrenocortical function in bronchial asthma." *Acta Medica Hungarica* (1983), 40(2–3):125–31.

Fitzsimmons, R., Grammar, L. C., et al. "Prevalence of adverse effects in corticosteroid dependent asthmatics." *New England and Regional Allergy Proceedings* (March–April 1988), 9(2):157–62.

Gluck, O. S., Murphy, W. A., et al. "Bone loss in adults receiving alternate day glucocorticoid therapy." *Arthritis and Rheumatology* (July 1981), 892–98.

Haffner, C. A., Kendall, M. J. "Metabolic effects of beta 2-agonists." *Journal of Clinical Pharmacology and Therapeutics* (June 1992), 17(3):155–64.

Karalus, N. C., Mahood, C. B., et al. "Adrenal function in acute severe asthma." *New Zealand Medical Journal* (Oct. 9, 1995), 98(788):843–46.

Knutsen, R., Bohmer, T., Falch, J. "Intravenous theophylline-induced excretion of calcium, magnesium and sodium in patients with recurrent asthmatic attacks." *Scandinavian Journal of Clinical and Laboratory Investigation* (April 1994), 54(2):119–25.

Lipworth, B. J., Clark, R. A. "The biochemical effects of high-dose inhaled salbutamol in patients with asthma." *European Journal of Clinical Pharmacology* (1989), 36(4):357–60.

Lofdahl, C. G., Svedmyr, N. "Beta-agonists: Friends or foes?" *European Respiratory Journal* (1991), 4:1161–65.

Luengo, M., Picado, C., et al. "Vertebral fractures in steroid dependent asthma and involutional osteoporosis: A comparative study." *Thorax* (November 1991), 46(11):803–06.

Nassif, E., Weinberger, M., et al. "Extrapulmonary effects of maintenance corticosteroid therapy with alternate-day prednisone and inhaled beclomethasone in children with chronic asthma." *Journal of Allergy and Clinical Immunology* (October 1987), 80(4):518–29.

Nicklas, R. A. "Paradoxical bronchospasm associated with the use of inhaled beta agonists." *Journal of Allergy and Clinical Immunology* (1990), 85:959–64.

Patterson, R., Walker, C. L., Greenberger, P. A., Sheridfan, E. P. "Prednisonephobia." *Allergy Proceedings* (November–December 1989), 10(6):423–28.

Pride, M., Deamer, R. L. "Over-the-counter cimetidine and theophylline interaction" (letter). *American Family Physician* (December 1995), 52(8):2180.

Scarfone, R. J., Loiselle, J. M., et al. "Nebulized dexamethasone versus oral prednisone in the emergency treatment of asthmatic children." *Annals of Emergency Medicine* (October 1995), 26(4):480–86.

Schiff, G. D., Hegde, H. K., Lacloche, L., Hryhorczuk, D. O. "Inpatient theophylline toxicity: Preventable factors." *Annals of Internal Medicine* (May 1991), 114(9):748–53.

Seneff, M., Scott, J., Friedman, B., Smith, M. "Acute theophylline toxicity and the use of esmolol to reverse cardiovascular instability." *Annals of Emergency Medicine* (June 1990), 19(6):671–73.

Sessler, C. N., Cohen, M. D. "Cardiac arrhythmias during theophylline toxicity. A prospective continuous electrocardiographic study." *Chest* (September 1990), 98(3): 672–78.

Shannon, M., Lovejoy, F. H., Jr., "The influence of age vs peak serum concentration on life-threatening events after chronic theophylline intoxication." *Archives of Internal Medicine* (October 1990), 150(10):2045–48.

Shields, M. D., Hicks, E. M., Macgregor, D. F., Richey, S. "Infantile spasms associated with theophylline toxicity." *Acta Paediatrica* (February 1995), 84(2):215–17.

Smith, B. J., Buxton, J. R., et al. "Does beclomethasone dipropionate suppress dehydroepiandrosterone sulphate in postmenopausal women?" *Australian and New Zealand Journal of Medicine* (August 1994), 24(4):396–401.

Spitzer, S. A., Kaufman, H., et al. "Beclomethasone dipropionate and chronic asthma. The effect of long-term aerosol administration on the hypothalamic-pituitary-adrenal axis after substitution for oral therapy with corticosteroids." *Chest* (July 1976), 70(1):38–42.

Spitzer, W. O., Suissa, S., et al. "The use of B-agonists and the risk of death and near death from asthma." *New England Journal of Medicine* (1992), 326:501–06.

Stein, M. A., Krasowski, M., Leventhal, B. L., Phillips, W., Bender, B. G. "Behavioral and cognitive effects of methylxanthines. A meta-analysis of theophylline and caffeine." *Archives of Pediatrics and Adolescent Medicine* (March 1996), 150(3):284–88.

Tinkelman, D. G., Moss, B. A., Bukantz, B. C., et al. "A multicenter trial of the prophylactic effect of ketotifen, theophylline, and placebo in atopic asthma." *Journal of Allergy and Clinical Immunology* (September 1985), 76(3):487–97.

Toogood, J. H., Markov, A. E., Baskerville, J., Dyson, C. "Association of ocular cataracts with inhaled and oral steroid therapy during long-term treatment of asthma." *Journal of Allergy and Clinical Immunology* (February 1993), 91(2):571–79.

Twentyman, O. P., Higenbottam, T. W. "Controversies in respiratory medicine: Regular inhaled beta-agonists—Clear clinical benefit or a hazard to health?" *Respiratory Medicine* (1992), 86(6):471–76.

Weinstein, R. E., Lobocki, C. A., et al. "Decreased adrenal sex steroid levels in the absence of glucocorticoid suppression in postmenopausal asthmatic women." *Journal of Allergy and Clinical Immunology* (January 1996), 97(1 Pt 1):1–8.

MAGNESIUM AND ASTHMA

Magnesium is known to play an important role in lung function. Studies show this mineral is deficient in many asthmatics, and replacement therapy is currently under evaluation. Numerous studies have shown its benefits.

Block, H., Silverman, R., Mancherje, N., Grant, S., Jagminas, L., Scharf, S. M. "Intravenous magnesium sulfate as an adjunct in the treatment of acute asthma." *Chest* (February 1990), 97(2):373–76.

Bloch, H., Silverman, R., et al. "Intravenous magnesium sulfate as an adjunct in the treatment of acute asthma." *Chest* (June 1995), 1576–81.

de Valk, H. W., Kok, P. T., Struyvenberg, A., van Rijn, H. J., Haalboom, J. R., Kreukniet, J., Lammers, J. W. "Extracellular and intracellular magnesium concentrations in asthmatic patients." *European Respiratory Journal* (September 1993), 6(8):1122–25.

Fantidis, P., Ruiz, Cacho, J., et al. "Intracellular polymorphonuclear magnesium content in patients with bronchial asthma between attacks." *Journal of the Royal Society of Medicine* (August 1995), 88(8):441–45.

Kok, P. T., Struyvenberg, A., et al. "Extracellular and intracellular magnesium concentration in asthmatic patients." *European Respiratory Journal* (September 1993), 1122–25.

Kuitert, L. M., Kletchko, S. L. "Intravenous magnesium sulfate in acute, life-threatening asthma." *Annals of Emergency Medicine* (November 1991), 1243–45.

Landon, R. A., Young, E. A. "Role of magnesium in regulation of lung function." *Journal of the American Dietetic Association* (June 1993), 93(6):674–77.

McLean, R. M. "Magnesium and its therapeutic uses: A review." *American Journal of Medicine* (January 1994), 96(1):63–76.

McNamara, R. M., Spivey, W. H., et al. "Intravenous magnesium sulfate in the management of acute respiratory failure complicating asthma." *Annals of Emergency Medicine* (February 1989), 197–99.

Manzke, H., Thiemeier, M., Elster, P., Lemke, J. "Magnesiumsulfat als Adjuvans bei der Inhalationstherapie des Asthma bronchiale mit Beta-2-Sympathikomimetika" (Magnesium sulfate as adjuvant in beta-2-sympathicomimetic inhalation therapy of bronchial asthma). *Pneumologie* (October 1990), 44(10):1190–92.

Mathew, R., Altura, B. M. "The role of magnesium in lung diseases: Asthma, allergy and pulmonary hypertension." *Magnesium and Trace Elements* (1991–92), 10(2–4):220–28.

Noppen, M., Vanmaele, L., et al. "Bronchodilating effect of intravenous magnesium sulfate in acute severe bronchial asthma." *Chest* (February 1990), 373–76.

Okayama, H., Aikawa, T., et al. "Bronchodilating effect of intravenous magnesium sulfate in bronchial asthma." *JAMA* (Feb. 27, 1987), 257(8):1076–78.

Rolla, G., Bucca, C., et al. "Reduction of histamine-induced bronchoconstriction by magnesium in asthmatic subjects." *Allergy* (April 1987), 42(3):186–88.

Skobeloff, E. M., Spivey, W. H., McNamara, R. M., Greenspon, L. "Intravenous magnesium sulfate for the treatment of acute asthma in the emergency department." *JAMA* (Sept. 1, 1989), 262(9):1210–13.

ENVIRONMENT AND ASTHMA

Our changing environment, both indoor and outdoor, is having a significant impact on asthmatic patients. Environmental toxins, ranging from formaldehyde to industrial soot and ozone, pose specific threats to the health of asthmatics.

Bardana, Emil J., Jr., Montanaro, Anthony, and O'Hollaren, Mark T. *Occupational Asthma*. Philadelphia: Hanley & Belfus, 1992.

Burge, P. S., Harries, M. G. "Occupational asthma due to formaldehyde." *Thorax* (April 1985), 40(4):255–60.

Cockcroft, D. W., Doeppner, V. H., Dolovich, J. "Occupational asthma caused by cedar urea formaldehyde particle board." *Chest* (June 1981):706–07.

Dadd, Debra Lynn. *The Nontoxic Home*. Los Angeles: Jeremy P. Tarcher, 1986.

Fairechild, Diana. *Jet Lag? Jet Smart*. Maui, Hawaii: Flyana Rhyme, 1992.

Frigas, E., Filley, W. V., Reed, C. E. "Asthma induced by dust from urea-formaldehyde foam insulating material." *Chest* (June 1981) 79(6):706–07.

Gannon, F., Bright, P., et al. "Occupational asthma due to glutaraldehyde and formaldehyde in endoscopy and X-ray departments." *Thorax* (February 1995), 50(2):156–59.

Gold, D. R. "Indoor air pollution." *Clinics in Chest Medicine* (June 1992), 13(2):215–19.

Golos, Natalie, O'Shea, James F., Waickman, Francis J., with Golbitz, Frances Golos. *Environmental Medicine*. New Canaan, CT: Keats Publishing, 1987.

Green, D. J., Saunder, L. R., et al. "Acute response to 3.0 ppm formaldehyde in exercising healthy nonsmokers and asthmatics." *American Review of Respiratory Disease* (June 1987), 1261–66.

Hayes, J. P. "Occupational asthma among hospital health care personnel: A cause for concern?" *Thorax* (1994), 198–200.

Rogers, Sherry A. *The E.I. Syndrome*. Syracuse, NY: Prestige Publishers, 1986.

Rousseau, David, Rea, W. J., and Enwright, Jean. *Your Home, Your Health, and Well-Being*. Vancouver: Hartley & Marks, 1989.

Schachter, E. N., Witek, T. J., Jr., et al. "A study of respiratory effects from exposure to 2.0 ppm formaldehyde in occupationally exposed workers." *Environmental Research* (December 1987), 188–205.

Stellman, Jeanne, and Henifin, Mary Sue. *Office Work Can Be Dangerous to Your Health*. New York: Random House, 1989.

Thrasher, J. D., Broughton, A., Madison, R. "Immune activation and autoantibodies in humans with long-term inhalation exposure to formaldehyde." *Archives of Environmental Health* (July–August 1980), 45:217–23.

Venolia, Carol. *Healing Environments*. Berkeley, CA: Celestial Arts, 1988.

Vidal, C., Gonzalez-Quintela, A. "Food-induced and occupational asthma due to barley flour." *Annals of Allergy, Asthma and Immunology* (August 1995), 75(2):121–24.

FOOD ALLERGIES, THE GASTROINTESTINAL TRACT AND ASTHMA

Food allergies can cause serious systemic effects in asthma patients, as well as more subtle symptoms. Food allergies can present an important avenue of evaluation in patients who do not respond to regular medical therapy, or in patients who experience erratic or unexplained asthma episodes.

Increased intestinal permeability may be due to inflammation in the gut lining, and may promote allergic reactions throughout the body, including asthma.

Antico, A. "Oral allergy syndrome induced by chestnut." *Annals of Allergy, Asthma and Immunology* (January 1996), 76(1):37–40.

Barrie, S. "Food Allergy" in *A Textbook of Natural Medicine* edited by J. E. Pizzorno and M. T. Murray. Seattle: John Bastyr College Publications, 1985.

Bjarnason, I., Ward, A., Peters, T. J. "The leaky gut of alcoholism: Possible root of entry for toxic compounds." *The Lancet* (Jan. 28, 1984), 179.

Boero, M., Pera, A., et al. "Candida overgrowth in gastric juice of peptic ulcer subjects on short- and long-term treatment with H2-receptor antagonists." *Digestion* (1983), 28(3):158–63.

Bousquet, J. "Mechanisms in adverse reactions to food. The lung." *Allergy* (1995), 50 (20 Suppl.), 52–55.

Brody, Jane E. "Beyond Ragweed: Allergenic Combinations." *New York Times*, Sept. 6, 1995, C10.

Buist, Robert. *Food Chemical Sensitivity*. Garden City, NY: Avery Publishing Group, 1988.

Businco, L., Falconieri, P., et al. "Food allergy and asthma." *Pediatric Pulmonology* supplement (1995), 11:59–60.

Dupont, C., Barau, E., et al. "Food induced alterations of intestinal permeability in children with cows' milk sensitivity, enteropathy and atopic dermatitis." *Journal of Pediatric Gastroenterology and Nutrition* (May 1989), 8(4):459–65.

Elia, M., Behrens, R., Northrop, C., et al. "Evaluation of mannitol, lactulose, and 51 Cr-EDTA as markers of intestinal permeability in man." *Clinical Science* 73 (1987), 197–204.

Heiner, Douglas, Wilson, John F. "Delayed immunologic food reactions." *NER Allergy Proceedings* (December 1986), 520–26.

Hemmings, W. A., Williams, E. W. "Transport of large breakdown products of dietary protein through the gut wall." *Gut* (August 1978), 19(8):715.

Herrmann, D., Henzgen, M., et al. "Effect of hyposensitization for tree pollinosis on associated apple allergy." *Journal of Investigational Allergology and Clinical Immunology* (September–October 1995), 5(5):259–67.

Hunter, J. O. "Food allergy—Or enterometabolic disorder?" *The Lancet* (Aug. 24, 1991), 495–96.

Malmgren, R., Unge, G., et al. "Lowered glutathione-peroxidase activity in asthmatic patients with food and aspirin intolerance." *Allergy* (January 1986), 43–45.

Miller, J. *Food Allergy, Provocative Testing and Injection Therapy*. Springfield, IL: Thomas, 1972.

Papageorgiou, Niki., Lee, T. H., et al. "Neutrophil chemotactic activity in milk-induced asthma." *Journal of Allergy and Clinical Immunology* (July 1983), 75–82.

Ratner, David, Shoshnai, Ehud, Dubnov, Boris. "Milk protein-free diet for nonseasonal asthma and migraine in lactase-deficient patients." *Israel Journal of Medical Sciences* (September 1983), 806–09.

Rinkel, H. J. "The diagnosis of food allergy." *Archives of Otolaryngology* 79 (1964), 71–79.

Sampson, Hugh, Mendelson, Louis, Rosen, James P. "Fatal and near-fatal anaphylactic reactions to food in children and adolescents." *New England Journal of Medicine* (August 1992), 380–44.

Tilles, S., Schocket, A., Milgrom, H. "Exercise-induced anaphylaxis related to specific foods." *Journal of Pediatric Allergy* (1995), 127:587–89.

HORMONES, DHEA AND ASTHMA

Hormones regulate numerous day-to-day body functions, and can affect asthma either through circadian (daily) variations or by acting as direct mediators in inflammation. Persons taking hormone replacement therapy should be aware that these hormones may worsen their condition.

DHEA is the most abundant adrenal hormone found in the body, and is a precursor for sex and other adrenal hormones. It has been shown to have benefit in certain inflammatory conditions such as lupus, and is currently being researched for a variety of other conditions, including asthma.

Dunn, P. J., Mahood, C. B., Speed, J. F., Jury, D. R. "Dehydroepiandrosterone sulphate concentrations in asthmatic patients: Pilot study." *New Zealand Journal of Medicine* (Nov. 28, 1984), 97(768):805–08.

Feher, K. G., Koo, E., Feher, T. "Adrenocortical function in bronchial asthma." *Acta Medica Hungarica* (1983), 40(2–3):125–31.

Lieberman, D., Kopernik, G., et al. "Sub-clinical worsening of bronchial asthma during estrogen replacement therapy in asthmatic post-menopausal women." *Maturitas* (February 1995), 21(2):153–57.

Smith, B. J., Buxton, J. R., Dickeson, J., Heller, R. F. "Does beclomethasone dipropionate suppress dehydroepiandrosterone sulphate in postmenopausal women?" *Australian and New Zealand Journal of Medicine* (August 1994), 24(4):396–401.

Troisi, R. J., Speizer, F. E., Willett, W. C., Trichopoulos, D., Rosner, B. "Menopause, postmenopausal estrogen preparations, and the risk of adult-onset asthma. A prospective cohort study." *American Journal of Respiratory and Critical Care Medicine* (October 1995), 152(4 Pt 1):1183–88.

Weinstein, R. E., Lobocki, C. A., Gravett, S., Hum, H., Negrich, R., Herbst, J., Greenberg, D., Pieper, D. R. "Decreased adrenal sex steroid levels in the absence of glucocorticoid suppression in postmenopausal asthmatic women." *Journal of Allergy and Clinical Immunology* (January 1996), 97(1 Pt 1):1–8.

NUTRIENTS AND ASTHMA

Specific nutrients are essential for normal function of the lung. Under stressful conditions, such as those produced during asthma attacks, intracellular deficiencies may occur. This may adversely affect asthma treatment. Supplementation can be beneficial and may augment other therapies.

An accumulating body of evidence points to the role of specific nutrients in health and disease. This is particularly important in treating asthma.

Abril, E. R., Rybski, J. A., et al. "Beta-carotene stimulates human leukocytes to secrete a novel cytokine." *Journal of Leukocyte Biology* (March 1989), 45(3):255–61.

Armstrong, P. L. "Iron deficiency in adolescents." *British Medical Journal* (Feb. 25, 1989), 298(6672):499.

Aruoma, O. I., Halliwell, B., et al. "The antioxidant action of N-acetylcysteine: Its reaction with hydrogen peroxide, hydroxyl radical, superoxide, and hypochlorous acid." *Free Radical Biologie Medicale* (1989), 6(6):593–97.

Bogden, J. D., Oleske, J. M., et al. "Zinc and immunocompetence in elderly people: Effects of zinc supplementation for 3 months." *American Journal of Clinical Nutrition* (September 1988), 48(3):655–63.

Calbom, Cherie, Keane, Maureen. *Juicing for Life: A Guide to the Health Benefits of Fresh Fruit and Vegetable Juicing.* Salt Lake City: Publishers Press, 1992, pp. 58–61.

Carper, Jean. *Jean Carper's Total Nutrition Guide.* New York: Bantam Books, 1989.

Chow, C. "Dietary vitamin E and cellular susceptibility to cigarette smoking." *Annals of the New York Academy of Science* (1982), 393.

Clark, A. J., Mossholder, S., Spengler, J. "Folacin status in adolescent females." *American Journal of Clinical Nutrition* (1987), 46:302–06.

Dawson-Hughes, B., Dallal, G. E., et al. "A controlled trial of the effect of calcium supplementation on bone density in postmenopausal women." *New England Journal of Medicine* (Sept. 27, 1990), 323(13):878–83.

Gey, K., Puska, P., et al. "Inverse correlation between plasma vitamin E and mortality from ischemic heart disease in cross-cultural epidemiology." *American Journal of Clinical Nutrition* (January 1991), 53(1 Suppl.):326S–334S.

Hasselmark, L., Malmgran, R., Zetterstrom, O., Unge, G. "Selenium supplementation in intrinsic asthma." *Allergy* (January 1993), 48(1):30–36.

Koop, C. E. —U.S. Department of Health and Human Services, Public Health Service. *The Surgeon General's Report on Nutrition and Health*, no. 88-50211. Washington, DC: Government Printing Office, 1988.

Levin, Buck. "Coenzyme Q: Clinical monograph." *Quarterly Review of Natural Medicine* (Fall 1994), 235–49.

Meydani, M., Macauley, J. B., Blumberg, J. B. "Effect of dietary vitamin E and selenium on susceptibility of brain region to lipid peroxidation." *Lipids* (1988), 23:405–09.

Pincemail, J., Deby, C. "The antiradical properties of Ginkgo Biloba extract." *Recent Results in Pharmacology and Clinic*, Springer-Verlag (1988), 71–82.

Prasad, A. S. "Clinical, biochemical and nutritional spectrum of zinc deficiency in human subjects: An update." *Nutrition Review* (1983), 41:197–208.

Schrauzer, G., Molenaar, T., et al. "Selenium in the blood of Japanese and American women with and without breast cancer and fibrocystic disease." *Japanese Journal of Cancer Research* (May 1985), 76(5):374–77.

Smith, Lewis J., Houston, M., Anderson, J. "Increased levels of glutathione in bronchoalveolar lavage fluid from patients with asthma." *American Review of Respiratory Disease* (1993), 1461–64.

Welton, A. F., Tobias, L. D., et al. "Effects of flavonoids on arachidonic acid metabolism." *Progress in Clinical Biological Residency* (1986), 213:231–32.

Wiseman, Helen. "Dietary influences on membrane function: Importance in protection against oxidative damage and disease." *Journal of Nutritional Biochemistry*, Elsevier Science (1996), 7(1):2–15.

BREATHING EXERCISES, BIOFEEDBACK, MEDITATION AND ASTHMA

Learning to breathe properly is an essential part of any asthma treatment program. Breathing exercises provide a powerful tool for overcoming asthma. Meditation, hypnosis, and other mind-body techniques can also be helpful in controlling the illness.

Aronoff, G. M., Aronoff, S., Peck, L. W. "Hypnotherapy in the treatment of bronchial asthma." *Annals of Allergy* (June 1975), 34(6):356–62.

David, Martha, Eshelman, Elizabeth Robbins, and McKay, Matthew. *The Relaxation and Stress Reduction Workbook*. Oakland, CA: New Harbinger Publications, 1988. Tape available from Vital Body Marketing, Manhasset, New York, 1990.

Epstein, Gerald. *Healing Visualizations*. New York: Bantam Books, 1989.

Goldman, Jonathan. *Healing Sounds: Power of Harmonics*. East Rutherford, NJ: Viking/Penguin, 1992.

Goyeche, J. R., Abo, Y., Ikemi, Y. "Asthma: The yoga perspective. Part II: Yoga therapy in the treatment of asthma." *Journal of Asthma* (1982), 19(3):189–201.

Green, Elmer and Alice. *Beyond Biofeedback*. New York: Delacorte Press/S. Lawrence, 1977.

Hobson, Allan. *The Chemistry of Conscious States: How the Brain Changes Its Mind*. Boston: Little, Brown, 1994.

Jain, S. C., Rai L., Valecha, A., Jha, U. K., Bhatnagar, S. O., Ram, K. "Effect of yoga training on exercise tolerance in adolescents with childhood asthma." *Journal of Asthma* (1991), 28(6):437–42.

Katz, R. M. "Asthma and sports." *Annals of Allergy* (August 1983), 51(2 Pt 1):153–60.

Leary, Warren E. "Study Induces Asthma Symptoms, Pointing to a Failure to Relax." *New York Times*, Nov. 1, 1995, C13.

Mellins, R. B. "Pulmonary physiotherapy in the pediatric age group." *American Review of Respiratory Disease* (December 1974), 110(6 Pt 2):137–42.

Morrison, J. B. "Chronic asthma and improvement with relaxation induced by hypnotherapy." *Journal of the Royal Society of Medicine* (December 1988), 701–04.

Rossi, Ernest Lawrence. *The Psychobiology of Mind-Body*. New York: W. W. Norton, 1986.

Scherr, M. S., Crawford, P. L., Sergent, C. B., Scherr, C. A. "Effect of bio-feedback techniques on chronic asthma in a summer camp environment." *Annals of Allergy* (November 1975), 35(5):289–95.

Singh, V., Wisniewski, A., Britton, J., Tattersfield, A. "Effect of yoga breathing exercises (pranayama) on airway reactivity in subjects with asthma" (see comments). *The Lancet* (June 9, 1990), 335(8702):1381–83.

Sorvino, Paul. *How to Become a Former Asthmatic.* New York: William Morrow & Co., 1985.

————. *How to Become a Former Asthmatic.* Tape of breathing exercises available from the Sorvino Asthma Foundation, 246 Lafayette Street, New York, NY 10012, 212-941-8686.

Stanescu, D. "Yoga breathing exercises and bronchial asthma" (letter; comment). *The Lancet* (Nov. 10, 1990), 336(8724):1192.

Thought Technology, 2180 Belgrave Avenue, Montreal, Quebec, Canada H4A 2L8 800-361-3651: Materials and equipment.

Tools for Exploration, 47 Paul Drive, San Rafael, CA 94903 800-456-9887: Breathwork explorer, biofeedback materials and supplies.

Weiner, P., Azgad, Y., Ganam, R., Weiner, M. "Inspiratory muscle training in patients with bronchial asthma." *Chest* (November 1992), 102(5):1357–61.

Wolf, S. I., Lampl, K. L. "Pulmonary rehabilitation: The use of aerobic dance as a therapeutic exercise for asthmatic patients." *Annals of Allergy* (November 1988), 61(5):357–60.

Young, S. H., Litz, S. "The Use of Hypnosis in the Treatment of Bronchial Asthma" in *Psychobiological Aspects of Allergic Disease,* edited by S. H. Young, J. Rubin, and H. Daman. Philadelphia: Prager, 1986.

GENERAL READING

Alternative Medicine the Definitive Guide, compiled by the Burton Goldberg Group. 3rd ed. Fife, WA: Future Medicine Publishing, 1994.

Arvigo, Rosita, and Balick, Michael. *Rainforest Remedies.* Twin Lakes, WI: Lotus Press, 1993.

Balch, Phyllis A., and Balch, James F. *Prescription for Dietary Wellness.* Greenfield, IN: PAB Books, 1992.

————. *Prescription for Nutritional Healing.* Garden City, NY: Avery Publishing Group, 1990.

Chopra, Deepak. *Perfect Health.* New York: Harmony Books, 1991.

Collinge, William. *The American Holistic Health Association Complete Guide to Alternative Health.* New York: Warner Books, 1996.

Delaney, Gayle. *Breakthrough Dreaming: How to Tap the Power of Your 24-Hour Mind.* New York: Bantam Books, 1991.

Eaton, S. B., Shostak, M., and Donner, M. *The Paleolithic Prescription: A Program of Diet and Exercise and a Design for Living.* New York: Harper & Row, 1988.

Giovannini, Marilyn. *The Complete Food Allergy Cookbook.* Rocklin, CA: Prima Publishing, 1996.

Hauri, Peter, and Linde, Shirley. *No More Sleepless Nights.* New York: John Wiley & Sons, 1991.

Hyde, J. S., and Swarts, C. L. "Effect of an exercise program on the perennially asthmatic child." *American Journal of Diseases of Children* (October 1968), 116(4):383–96.

Jelks, Mary, *Allergy Plants That Cause Sneezing and Wheezing.* Tampa, FL: Worldwide Printing, 1991.

Maharam, Lewis G. *The Exercise High.* New York: Ballantine Books, 1992.

Massey, L. K., and Strang, M. "Soft drink consumption, phosphorus intake, and osteoporosis." *Journal of the American Dietetic Association* 80 (1982), 581.

Moyers, Bill. *Healing and the Mind.* New York: Doubleday, 1993.

Murray, Michael, and Pizzorno, Joseph. *Encyclopedia of Natural Medicine.* Rocklin, CA: Prima Publishing, 1991.

Odey, Penelope. *The Complete Medicinal Herbal.* New York: Dorling Kindersley, 1993.

Pahlow, Mannfried. *Healing Plants.* English translation available from Barron's Educational Series, Inc. Hauppauge, NY: 1993.

Plebani, M., Borghesan, F., and Faggian, D. "Clinical efficiency of in vitro and in vivo tests for allergic diseases." *Annals of Allergy, Asthma and Immunology* (January 1995), 74(1):23–28.

Pollen Guide. Round Rock, TX: Meridian Bio-Medical, 1991.

Randolph, T. G. and Moss, R. W. *An Alternative Approach to Allergies.* New York: HarperCollins, 1990.

Reuben, Carolyn. *Antioxidants. Your Complete Guide.* Rocklin, CA: Prima Publishing, 1995.

Salaman, Maureen, and Scheer, James F. *Foods That Heal.* Menlo Park, CA: M.K.S., Inc., 1994.

Shama, H. M., Triguna, B. D., and Chopra, D. "Maharishi Ayur-veda: Modern insights into ancient medicine." *Journal of the American Medical Association* 265 (20) (May 22, 29, 1991), 2633–37.

Siegel, Bernie S. *Peace, Love and Healing. Bodymind Communication and the Path of Self-healing: An Exploration.* New York: Harper & Row, 1989.

Smith, B. "Organic foods vs supermarket foods: Element levels." *Journal of Applied Nutrition* 45 (1993), 35–39.

Trattler, Ross. *Better Health Through Natural Healing.* New York: McGraw-Hill Book Company, 1985.

Tsuei, J. J., Lehman, C. W., et al. "A food allergy study utilizing the EAV acupuncture technique." *American Journal of Acupuncture* 12 (1984), 105–16.

Weil, Andrew. *Spontaneous Healing.* New York: Alfred A. Knopf, 1995.

Whitaker, Julian. *Dr. Whitaker's Guide to Natural Healing.* Rocklin, CA: Prima Publishing, 1995.

Winter, Ruth. *A Consumer's Dictionary of Food Additives.* 4th ed. New York: Crown paperback, 1994.

Young, S. H., Dobozin, B., and Minor, M. *The Consumers Complete Guide to Allergy.* New York: Consumer Reports Publishing, 1992.

Young, S. H., Shulman, S., and Shulman, M. *The Asthma Handbook.* 2nd ed. New York: Bantam Books, 1989.

INDEX